ANTIBODY APPLICATIONS

ESSENTIAL TECHNIQUES SERIES

Series Editor
D. Rickwood
Department of Biology, University of Essex, Wivenhoe Park, Colchester, UK

Published titles
Antibody Applications
Gel Electrophoresis: Nucleic Acids

Forthcoming titles
PCR
Gene Transcription
Human Chromosome Preparation
Protein Gel Electrophoresis

ANTIBODY APPLICATIONS
ESSENTIAL TECHNIQUES

Peter J. Delves

Department of Immunology, UCL Medical School, London, UK

JOHN WILEY & SONS

Chichester • New York • Brisbane • Toronto • Singapore

Published in association with BIOS Scientific Publishers Limited

© BIOS Scientific Publishers Limited, 1995. Published by John Wiley & Sons Ltd, Baffins Lane, Chichester, West Sussex PO19 1UD, UK, in association with BIOS Scientific Publishers Ltd, 9 Newtec Place, Magdalen Road, Oxford OX4 1RE, UK.

British Library Cataloguing in Publication Data
A catalogue record for this book is available from the British
Library.

ISBN 0 471 95698 8

Typeset by Herb Bowes Graphics, Oxford, UK
Printed and bound in UK by Biddles Ltd, Guildford, UK

CONTENTS

ABBREVIATIONS

AP	alkaline phosphatase
APAAP	alkaline phosphatase–anti-alkaline phosphatase
BAC-SulfoNHS	biolinamidocaproate-*N*-hydroxysulfosuccinimide ester
BCIG	5-bromo-4-chloro-3-indolyl-β-D-galacto-pyranoside
BCIP	5-bromo-4-chloro-3-indolylphosphate
BSA	bovine serum albumin
BSS	balanced salt solution
CMC	carboxymethyl cellulose
DAB	diaminobenzidine
DABCO	1,4-diazobicyclo-[2.2.2]-octane
DEAE	diethylaminoethyl cellulose
DMSO	dimethylsulfoxide
EBV	Epstein–Barr virus
ELISA	enzyme-linked immunosorbent assay
FACS	fluorescent-activated cell sorter
FCS	fetal calf serum
FITC	fluorescein isothiocyanate
HGPRT	hypoxanthine guanine phosphoribosyl transferase
HIFCS	heat-inactivated fetal calf serum
HRP	horseradish peroxidase
IEF	isoelectric focusing
IPTG	isopropyl β-D-thiogalactopyranoside
MAb	monoclonal antibody
NBT	nitro blue tetrazolium
PAGE	polyacrylamide gel electrophoresis
PAP	peroxidase–anti-peroxidase
PBS	phosphate-buffered saline
PE	phycoerythrin
PMSF	phenylmethylsulfonyl fluoride
pNPP	*p*-nitrophenyl phosphate
RIA	radioimmunoassay
RT	room temperature
SAC	*Staphylococcus aureus* Cowan 1
SCID	severe combined immunodeficiency
SDS	sodium dodecyl sulfate, sodium lauryl sulfate
SRBC	sheep red blood cells
TBS	Tris-buffered saline
TEMED	tetramethylethylenediamine
TK	thymidine kinase
TMB	tetramethylbenzidine
TR	Texas red
TRITC	tetramethylrhodamine isothiocyanate

PREFACE

This book is intended to provide a simple step by step guide for those antibody-based and associated techniques which are most commonly used by both researchers and students. Protocols are not provided for some of the more specialized applications nor for the production of antibodies.

The protocols herein should give satisfactory and reproducible results in a variety of situations and I have tried to make them accessible to novices. The right hand side of each protocol contains blank space for the reader to add their own notes, and also contains annotations for some of the individual steps in the protocols, together with an indication of hazards associated with each step and at which points the protocol may be halted.

I would like to thank Jonathan Ray and Jane Campbell at BIOS, and the series editor David Rickwood, for their friendly help and advice during the preparation of the manuscript.

Peter J. Delves

SAFETY

Attention to safety aspects is an integral part of all laboratory procedures and national legislations impose legal requirements on those persons planning or carrying out such procedures. While the author, editor, and publisher believe that the recipes and practical procedures, as set forth in this book, are in accord with current recommendations and practice at the time of publication, they accept no legal responsibility for any errors or omissions, and make no warranty, expressed or implied, with respect to material contained herein. It remains the responsibility of the reader to ensure that the procedures which are followed are carried out in a safe manner and that all necessary safety instructions and national regulations are implemented.

In view of ongoing research, equipment modifications and changes in governmental regulations, the reader is urged to review and evaluate the information provided by the manufacturer, for each reagent, piece of equipment or device, for any changes in the instructions or usage and for added warnings and precautions.

All procedures mentioned within this book must be carried out under conditions of good laboratory practice in accordance with local and national guidelines. Some procedures involve specific hazards, including but not limited to, hazards in the following categories:

Other safety information on the Internet can be accessed on:

gopher://atlas.chem.utah.edu/11/MSDS
gopher://ginfo.cs.fit.edu:70/lm/safety/msds
http://physchem.ox.ac.uk/MSDS
http://www.fisher1.com/Fischer/Alphabetical Index.html
http://www.pp.orst.edu

You are actively encouraged to check these data sheets to confirm our assignments and for more detailed information on individual hazards; however the author, editor and publisher can accept no responsibility for any material contained in these data sheets. Furthermore, you must always follow the precautions outlined on labels and data sheets provided by individual manufacturers.

Radiation. The use of radioisotopes is subject to legislation and requires permission in most countries. Furthermore, national guidelines for their use and disposal must be rigorously adhered to. The procedures in protocols that use radioisotopes must only be carried out by individuals who have received training in the use of such material using the appropriate facilities, protection and personal monitoring procedures.

Biological. Antibodies, sera and cells (particularly, but not exclusively, those of human and non-human primate origin) pose

Chemical. A number of the reagents are known to be carcinogenic, mutagenic, toxic, inflammable, highly reactive or otherwise hazardous. Substances known to be hazardous have been marked with the symbol ⚠ in the list of reagents (but not subsequently) for each protocol, or if they appear as alternatives to the main protocol, the *first time* they appear in the notes. The reader should consult the safety notes on these pages before embarking on any of the procedures covered. This is in no way meant to imply that undesignated chemicals are non-hazardous, and all laboratory chemicals should be handled with extreme caution. Information is not available on the possible hazards of many compounds. The criteria we have generally used for denoting a substance with ⚠ is based upon a hazard level of 2 or more (on a scale 0–4) in any of the categories in the Baker Saf-T-Data™ system used in the material safety data sheets (MSDS) held at the University of Oxford, UK. These are freely accessible using:

http://joule.pcl.ox.ac.uk/MSDS/.

a significant biological hazard. All such materials, whatever their origin, may harbor human pathogens and should be handled as potentially infectious material in accordance with local guidelines. Any recombinant DNA work associated with protocols is likely to require permission from the relevant regulatory body and you must consult your local safety officer before embarking upon this work.

Electrical. Many of the procedures in this book use electrical equipment. Electrophoresis techniques may present particular hazards of this nature.

Lasers. Flow cytometers and certain other types of laboratory equipment contain lasers. Users should ensure they are fully aware of the potential hazards of using such equipment.

Antibody production

Antibodies secreted *in vivo* in response to immunization with antigen are usually polyclonal because several different B-cells will be stimulated which recognize different epitopes on the immunogen. Antisera can be raised in a wide range of animals [1]. Usually two or more injections of the antigen are given with adjuvant (a nonspecific enhancer of the immune response) and, for small molecules, a carrier (which provides determinants recognized by helper T-cells). Upon repeated immunization the antibodies produced will be mostly IgG, usually of a reasonably high affinity. The antiserum may require absorption to remove unwanted specificities. In contrast, an antibody molecule derived from a single clone of B-cells is referred to as a monoclonal antibody. Each antibody molecule secreted by the clone will have an identical polypeptide sequence and antigen-binding specificity. Monoclonal antibodies are most readily produced using the hybridoma technique of Köhler and Milstein [2, 3]. Lymphocytes from an immunized animal are mixed with a myeloma cell line (B-cell tumor) in the presence of a fusogenic reagent, usually polyethylene glycol. Myeloma cell lines which do not secrete immunoglobulin are usually chosen so that a single species of antibody molecule will be produced, that is that from the normal tumor) B-cell. The hybrid cell (hybridoma) inherits antigen specificity from the normal B-cell, and immortality from the tumor B-cell. Unfused normal B-cells are not immortal and die in culture. The myeloma cell lines used are mutants selected for lack of the enzymes hypoxanthine guanine phosphoribosyl transferase (HGPRT) and thymidine kinase (TK) and they are unable to use the salvage pathways of nucleic acid synthesis. The mutant myeloma therefore dies if the principal pathway for purine and pyrimidine synthesis is blocked using the folic acid analog aminopterin, since neither pathway is then available to it. The hybridoma, however, inherits the salvage pathway genes from the normal B-cell and is able to utilize hypoxanthine and thymidine, thus surviving in 'HAT' medium (hypoxanthine, aminopterin, thymidine) [4–7].

Hybridoma cells can be 'cloned' by seeding them at an average of <1 cell/well in 96-well microtiter plates containing irradiated feeder cells [8]. Usually all the cells that grow in a well will be identical because they have been derived from a single cell. By repeating this limiting dilution two or three times, a clone can be obtained which can then be continuously grown in tissue culture, and the supernatants harvested for isolation of the secreted monoclonal antibody. Sometimes these hybridomas are not very stable over long-term culture periods, but one can insure against this by freezing down aliquots of the hybridoma in liquid nitrogen which can then be used to start fresh cultures secreting the same monoclonal antibody. For commercial production of monoclonal antibodies the cells can be grown in bioreactors which allow the cells to grow at high densities (e.g. 10^8/ml) whilst actively secreting large amounts (several grams/week) of antibody [9].

Human B-cells can be immortalized using the Epstein–Barr virus (EBV) and cloned to produce human monoclonal antibodies [10]. Whilst this technique is often employed successfully, it is also frequently observed that cells that grow out from these cultures lose their ability to secrete antibody after a period in culture, have a low cloning efficiency, and do not secrete high levels of antibody. However, EBV transformation can be followed by fusion with a myeloma cell line, thus allowing higher levels of antibody production and improved stability [11]. There is still no ideal human fusion partner for human B-cells; human myelomas grow poorly in culture and human lymphoblastoid cell lines generally show a low fusion frequency and secrete endogenous antibody [12]. Attempts to overcome this problem have involved the use of heterohybridomas in which the human B-cell is fused with a murine myeloma cell line, or even with a heteromyeloma which is itself a fusion of a murine and a human myeloma cell line [13]. However, such heterohybridomas suffer from chromosomal instability, although this is less pronounced when using a heteromyeloma partner. There is also the problem of being unable, for ethical reasons, to immunize human subjects with most antigens. Without prior immunization, the chances of obtaining high affinity monoclonal antibodies is remote. More recent approaches utilize immunization of severe combined immunodeficient (SCID) mice which have been reconstituted with a human immune system [14], immunization of mice transgenic for germ line human Ig gene segments (e.g. HuMAb-mouse™ from GenPharm International, Mountain View, CA) which undergo rearrangement upon B-cell differentiation [15], and direct cloning of rearranged Ig genes for phage display [16, 17] followed by mutagenesis [18] or chain shuffling [19] approaches in order to improve the affinity of the antibodies.

The choice between monoclonal or polyclonal antibodies

Monoclonal antibodies provide reagents with a single epitope specificity and potentially limitless amounts of identical antibody. On the other hand, polyclonal antibodies contain multiple specificities and are limited in quantity to the amount of serum that can be obtained from the immune animal. However, with medium sized species, such as a rabbit, enough serum (up to 80 ml) can be obtained from a hyperimmunized individual to yield high titer antibodies which will last, for most applications, for several years. Even from a mouse it is possible to obtain up to 1.5 ml of serum, which with a high titer antibody used at, for example, 1:10 000, would provide 15 liters of working strength antibody! Paradoxically, polyclonal antibodies can sometimes provide greater specificity than a monoclonal antibody against the same antigen. This is because undesirable cross-reactions can be removed from a polyclonal serum by absorption with the offending antigen, whereas any unwanted cross-reactions cannot be removed from a monoclonal antibody because there is only a single specificity. The specificity of polyclonal antibodies can also be improved by affinity chromatography using purified antigen.

Antibody fragments

It is sometimes desirable to avoid Fc-mediated effector functions of antibodies [20], such as binding to cellular Fc receptors when wishing to detect cell surface antigens. This can be achieved by digestion of the antibody with proteolytic enzymes [21, 22]. Cleavage with pepsin produces F(ab')$_2$ fragments which can then be separated from Fc fragments and any remaining undigested antibody using protein A or protein G-Sepharose chromatography. Alternatively, papain digestion will generate monovalent Fab fragments [23, 24].

Storage of antibodies

Antibodies can be stored in several different buffers at neutral pH but are most commonly kept in 0.01 M phosphate-buffered saline (PBS) pH 7.4 containing 0.1% sodium azide to inhibit microbial growth. In order to change a buffer, proteins should be dialyzed against several changes of the new buffer. A very quick and simple alternative method is desalting on a PD-10 column containing Sephadex G-25 (PD-10 columns are available from Pharmacia pre-packed with Sephadex G-25). For long-term storage, antibodies should be kept at –20°C or –70°C, although the colder temperature is usually not necessary. They should be stored at >0.5 mg/ml or in the presence of a carrier protein, for example 1% bovine serum albumin (BSA). If stored frozen, avoid freeze/thawing by making a number of aliquots and keeping each individual aliquot at 4°C subsequent to thawing. Aliquots of precious sera should be stored in two different freezers if possible, to insure against freezer breakdown. Antibodies kept at 4°C should either be sterile filtered through a 0.22-μm pore size Millipore filter, or kept in the presence of 0.1% sodium azide. It is extremely difficult to filter sterilize concentrated proteins (e.g. neat serum) and these should be diluted before filtration in order to facilitate this process. A first filtration through a 0.45-μm pore size membrane will also make filtration through the smaller pore size easier. Antibody conjugates are usually stored at 4°C but may also be stored at –20°C in 50% glycerol.

Whilst antibodies *in vivo* are catabolized within a matter of days or weeks, antibodies stored under the above conditions in the laboratory will remain immunologically active for several years. Antigen-binding activity of antibodies stored frozen for >10 years will usually still show acceptable binding as long as they have not been thawed out due to freezer breakdown, power supply interruptions, and so forth.

It is sometimes recommended that antibodies should be spun in a microfuge at 16 000 g in order to remove aggregates. This procedure will only bring down very large aggregates. If it is important to remove aggregates, for example where binding to Fc receptors may occur, this should be done by centrifugation at 120 000 g for 15 min in an ultracentrifuge.

Complement inactivation

The lytic complement activity of serum can be abolished by heating at 56°C for 30 min. In order to avoid denaturation of the antibody it is important not to exceed this temperature.

Antibody–antigen equilibrium

Although antibody binding to antigen can be detected within seconds, equilibrium is not usually reached until several hours after addition of antibody to antigen. For most assay purposes, however, incubations of 1–2 h will yield near maximal binding. The rate is affected by temperature, and therefore shorter incubation times should be carried out at 37°C whilst longer incubations (e.g. overnight) can be carried out at 4°C. The term room temperature (RT) is used throughout this book to denote a temperature of approximately 20°C.

Making dilutions

Make up dilutions of each reagent before use. For example, if 10 wells in a microtiter plate each need a 1 in 100 dilution of antibody added to them, do not add 99 μl buffer/well then 1 μl antibody/well, but make up 1 in 100 antibody first and then aliquot out 100 μl into each well. This will eliminate errors in the dilution between different wells (but not errors in pipetting into each well). Always make up approximately 10% more reagent than required for losses on the walls of the tube, etc. It is a sensible ploy always to glance at the pipette tip when taking up reagents to check that approximately the expected amount has been taken up. With experience, it becomes known where, for example, 100 μl reaches in the tip. If tips are not fastened securely enough to achieve an air-tight seal, or if the end of the pipette becomes scratched, the pipette may not take up the required volume. This is one of the most common reasons for poor immunoassay duplicates. Pipettes should be used in accordance with the manufacturer's instructions, and checked regularly for damage and accuracy.

Titration of antibodies

The titer of an antibody refers to the lowest concentration (highest dilution) of antibody that is still effective in a given assay system, for example agglutination. This is not the same as the working dilution which is usually a concentration which gives a good sensitivity with a high signal:noise ratio. Antibodies must therefore be titrated before use in any immunoassay system because use at too high a concentration is extremely wasteful, can give rise to a nonspecific signal in direct binding assays, and will be insensitive in inhibition assays. Conversely, too low a concentration will obviously lead to a loss in sensitivity.

In assays where the binding of a primary antibody is detected using a labeled secondary antibody (enzyme-linked immunosorbent assay (ELISA), radioimmunoassay (RIA), immunofluorescence, immunohistochemistry, etc.) titration is most conveniently carried out by setting up a criss-cross analysis to determine simultaneously the optimal dilution of both antibodies. In the ELISA example shown below a fourfold dilution series is shown for the primary antibody and a twofold dilution series for the secondary antibody in a 96-well microtiter plate carried out in duplicate. For assays which are not themselves carried out in microtiter plates, the dilutions can also be made in a microtiter plate or can be made in tubes. The titration should be carried out using both the relevant antigen/cells/tissue and an irrelevant antigen/cells/tissue. The aim is to establish dilutions which show strong binding to the relevant target, and no or very low binding to the irrelevant control. It is often necessary to repeat the titration experiment, using a wide range of dilutions the first time round to get an approximate figure and then using a narrower range of concentrations to improve it. If using commercially obtained antibodies the working dilution specified by the manufacturers can be used, although it is often worthwhile carrying out a titration to optimize their use in individual assay systems.

Table 1. Antibody titration for ELISA

	1	2	3	4	5	6	7	8	9	10	11	12	Dilutions of secondary antibody
A	over	over	over	over	2.500	2.500	2.419	2.421	1.001	0.099	0.040	0.042	1:20
B	over	over	over	over	2.420	2.420	2.409	2.407	0.087	0.088	0	0	1:40
C	over	over	2.469	2.472	2.307	2.311	1.989	1.991	0.064	0.062	0	0	1:80
D	2.498	2.488	2.100	2.101	1.710	1.710	1.101	1.436	0.021	0.025	0	0	1:160
E	1.546	1.541	1.333	1.326	1.178	1.179	0.888	0.891	0	0	0	0	1:320
F	0.765	0.769	0.212	0.212	0.065	0.067	0.010	0.004	0	0	0	0	1:640
G	0.100	0.099	0.032	0.037	0.001	0.004	0	0	0	0	0	0	1:1280
H	0	0	0	0	0	0	0	0	0	0	0	0	1:2560
	1:250		1:1 000		1:4 000		1:16 000		1:64 000		1:256 000		

Dilutions of primary antibody

In the example given (*Table 1*), the optimal dilutions to use would be 1:16 000 for the primary antibody, and 1:40 for the secondary antibody, assuming that there was no significant binding to the control antigen at these dilutions. The primary antibody could probably be used at less than 1:16 000 and a second titration could be carried out using dilutions between 1:10 000 and 1:50 000. Note that the duplicates are usually very close in this experiment except in row D, columns 7 and 8. The most likely cause would be a pipetting error. Overall, the primary antibody has a moderate titer but the secondary antibody has a low titer in this system.

Standard curves

In assays which are aimed at the quantification of a ligand of unknown concentration, a binding curve should be constructed using known concentrations of the protein. This is most easily achieved by making sequential dilutions (e.g. twofold, fourfold or tenfold) from a preparation of known concentration. The values obtained in the assay system (e.g. optical density) can then be plotted against the concentration of ligand (see *Figure 1*).

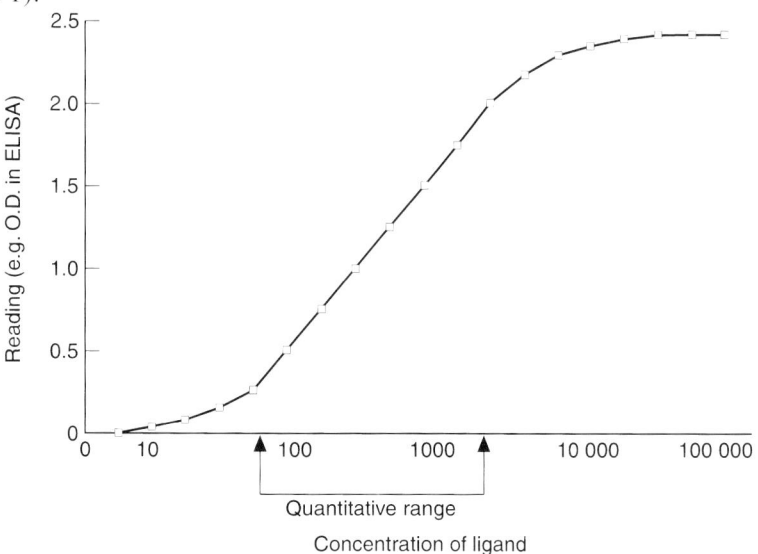

Figure 1. The binding curve is quantitative for those concentrations lying on the linear exponential portion of the graph.

General introduction

Kits

For many techniques pre-assembled kits are available. These kits include most or all of the reagents required for a particular procedure together with a booklet describing the protocol. The advantage is that everything has been quality controlled, and that the technique is made as simple as possible for those inexperienced in a particular method. The major disadvantage is cost, particularly as it is frequently the case that, for the application of choice, one of the reagents in the kit is used up well before the others.

Characterization of antibodies

Whilst it is intended that this book deals with antibody applications, many of the protocols provided cover assay systems which are also used for the characterization of antibodies. The major characteristics of an antibody molecule, which are desirable to establish, are the class of heavy and light chain, the antigen specificity, the epitope specificity, and the affinity.

(i)   The class and subclass can be determined with antibodies which are specific for the individual isotypes, using almost any system which measures reactivity of an antibody with antigen (in this case the antigen is the antibody to be characterized; see protocols for RIA, ELISA, double immunodiffusion, single radial immunodiffusion and crossed immunoelectrophoresis).

(ii) The antigen which the antibody was raised against will usually be known (if it is not then determining the specificity will require an enormous degree of luck) but its cross-reactivity with other antigens may not be known. It is a particularly common problem that 'species-specific' anti-immunoglobulins may in fact cross-react with immunoglobulins from other species. It is important to ascertain that in the system you intend to use the antibody does not show undesirable cross-reactions. This can be done by screening against relevant panels of antibodies, antigens and/or tissues (see protocols for RIA, ELISA, double immunodiffusion, immuno-fluorescence, immunohistochemistry).

(iii) If more than one monoclonal antibody against an antigen of interest is available, it is often desirable to determine if they recognize the same or different epitopes on the antigen [25, 26]. For example, if two monoclonal antibodies are to be used in a sandwich assay they must recognize different epitopes. This screening process can be done using an inhibition ELISA (*Protocol 9*) and/or two-site (sandwich) ELISA (*Protocol 7*). If novel specificities are revealed using this approach, it might be of interest to further define the epitope recognized. For continuous linear epitopes this can be carried out using the PEPSCAN™ system. Linear epitopes can also be displayed as libraries on the surface of bacteriophage [27]. For discontinuous epitopes there are several options available but none of them is particularly straightforward. Fragments of the antigen can be generated from the protein using, for example, proteolytic enzyme cleavage or recombinant DNA techniques, and the reactivity of the monoclonal antibodies (MAbs) with the fragments tested using ELISA and/or immunoblotting. Where sequences are relatively well conserved between species, the binding of MAbs to a panel of the antigens purified from the different species can be carried out and the results analyzed in the light of the published sequences. Recombinant DNA techniques can further be used to mutate individual amino acids and thus further help define the epitope [28].

(iv) The affinity of an antibody can be difficult to measure accurately, particularly as the value obtained varies somewhat depending upon the method used. However, most methods do provide a way of ranking antibodies in terms of their relative affinities and an ELISA of the type described in *Protocol 8* can be used to provide an estimate of antibody affinity [29].

References

1. Thanavala, Y. (1992) in *Encyclopedia of Immunology* (I.M. Roitt and P.J. Delves, eds), pp. 153–155. Academic Press, London.
2. Köhler, G. and Milstein, C. (1975) *Nature* **256**, 495–497.
3. Köhler, G. and Milstein, C. (1976) *Eur. J. Immunol.* **6**, 511–519.
4. Goding, J.W. (1986) *Monoclonal antibodies: Principles and Practice,* 2nd Edn. Academic Press, San Diego.
5. Liddell, J.E. and Cryer, A. (1991) *A Practical Guide to Monoclonal Antibodies.* John Wiley and Sons, Chichester.
6. Peters, J.H. and Baumgarten, H. (eds) (1992) *Monoclonal Antibodies.* Springer-Verlag, New York.
7. Yelton, D.E. and Scharff, M.D. (1981) *Annu. Rev. Biochem.* **50**, 657–680.
8. Ozaki, S. (1994) in *Cellular Immunology Labfax* (P.J. Delves, ed.), pp. 65–93. BIOS Scientific Publishers, Oxford.
9. Prior, C.P. (1991) in *Animal Cell Bioreactors,* (C.S. Ho and D.I.C. Wang, eds), pp. 445–478. Butterworth-Heinemann, Boston.
10. Steinmetz, M., Klein, G., Koskimies, S. and Makela, O. (1977) *Nature* **269**, 420–422.
11. Kozbor, D., Lagarde, A.E. and Roder, J.C. (1982) *Proc. Natl Acad. Sci. USA* **79**, 6651–6655.
12. Hohmann, A.W., Spatz, L., Irigoyen, M. and Manheimer-Lory, A. (1995) in *Monoclonal Antibodies: The Second Generation.* (H. Zola, ed.), pp. 43–66. BIOS Scientific Publishers, Oxford.
13. Kozbor, D., Tripputi, P., Roder, J.C. and Croce, C.M. (1984) *J. Immunol.* **133**, 3001–3005.

14. Duchosal, M.A., Eming, S.A., Fischer, P. *et al.* (1992) *Nature* **355**, 258–262.
15. Lonberg, N., Taylor, L.D., Harding, F.A. *et al.* (1994) *Nature* **368**, 856–859.
16. McCafferty, J., Griffiths, A.D., Winter, G. and Chiswell, D.J. (1990) *Nature* **348**, 552–554.
17. Borrebaeck, C.A.K. (ed.) (1992) *Antibody Engineering: a Practical Guide.* W.H. Freeman and Co, New York.
18. Gram, H., Marconi, L.-A., Barbas, C.F. III, Collet, T.A., Lerner, R.A. and Kang, A.S. (1992) *Proc. Natl Acad. Sci. USA* **89**, 3576–3580.
19. Marks, J.D., Griffiths, A.D., Malmqvist, M., Clackson, T., Bye, J.M. and Winter, G. (1992) *Bio/Technology* **10**, 779–783.
20. Morgan, E.L. and Weigle, W.O. (1987) *Adv. Immunol.* **40**, 61–134.
21. Porter, R.R. (1959) *Biochem. J.* **73**, 119–126.
22. Porter, R.R. (1973) *Science* **180**, 713–716.
23. Davies, M.E., Barrett, A.J. and Hembry, R.M. (1978) *J. Immunol. Methods* **21**, 305–315.
24. Kerr, M.A., Loomes, L.M. and Thorpe, S.J. (1994) in *Immunochemistry Labfax* (M.A. Kerr and R. Thorpe, eds), pp. 83–114. BIOS Scientific Publishers, Oxford.
25. Bidart, J.M., Troalen, F., Lazar, V., Berger, P., Marcillac, I., Lhomme, C., Droz, J.P. and Bellet, D. (1992) *Endocrinology*, **131**, 1832–1840.
26. Becker, S., Armbruster, F.P., Muller, B., Echner, H., Kapurnotu, A., Livaniou, E., Mihelic, M., Stoeva, S. and Voelter, W. (1994) *J. Immunol. Methods* **177**, 131–137.
27. Folgori, A., Tafi, R., Meola, A., Felici, F., Galfre, G., Cortese, R., Monaci, P. and Nicosia, A. (1994) *EMBO J.* **9**, 2236–2243.
28. Prasad, L., Sharma, S., Vandonselaar, M., Quail, J.W., Lee, J.S., Waygood, E.B., Wilson, K.S., Dauter, Z. and Delbaere, L.T.J. (1993) *J. Biol. Chem.* **268**, 10705–10708.
29. Friguet, B., Chaffotte, A.F., Djavadi-Ohaniance, L. and Goldberg, M.E. (1985) *J. Immunol. Methods* **77**, 305–319.

II LABELING OF ANTIBODIES

There are two major ways in which the binding of an antibody to an antigen is commonly visualized. Antibodies are at least bivalent and when they react with multivalent antigens there is the possibility of generating immune complexes that precipitate out of solution to form a visible pellet following centrifugation, produce a band or ring of precipitation in a gel, or agglutinate a particulate antigen. Many of these traditional immunoprecipitation and agglutination techniques continue to find a place in modern day research. An alternative, and more widely applicable approach, is to label the antibody (or antigen) with a molecule that can be readily detected. Most frequently these are enzymes, fluorochromes, radioisotopes or ligands for other labeled molecules. Although the antibody which binds to the specific antigen of interest (i.e. the primary antibody) is sometimes labeled, indirect techniques are more versatile. These involve using a labeled secondary antibody which is specific for the primary antibody (i.e. a labeled anti-immunoglobulin). This approach has the major advantage that only a single reagent needs to be labeled rather than having to conjugate every antibody that is to be tested. An additional advantage is that amplification of the signal can be achieved if a labeled polyclonal anti-immunoglobulin is used, because there is the potential for more than one molecule to bind to the primary antibody.

Methods available

Enzyme labeling (see *Protocol 2*)
Enzymes which cause a color change in a substrate are usually chosen, most frequently horseradish peroxidase or alkaline phosphatase. These are the most popular type of label for immunoassays due to the ease of the labeling procedure and stability of the labeled antibody. Qualitative detection can be achieved simply by visual inspection, whereas quantitative immunoassay measurements require an ELISA plate reader. For immuno-

References

1. Nakane, P.K. and Pierce, G.B. Jr (1967) *J. Cell Biol.* **33**, 307–318.
2. Scouten, W.H. (1987) *Methods Enzymol.* **135**, 30–65.
3. Tijssen, P. and Kurstak, E. (1984) *Anal. Biochem.* **136**, 451–457.
4. Greenwood, F.C., Hunter, W.M. and Glover, J.S. (1963) *Biochem. J.* **89**,114–123.
5. McConahey, P.J. and Dixon, F.J. (1980) *Methods Enzymol.* **70**, 210–213.

histochemistry and membrane-based assays a substrate which forms an insoluble product is used [1–3].

Problems: Some tissues contain endogenous enzyme activities which lead to high backgrounds. Some substrates may be carcinogenic.

Radiolabeling (see *Protocol 3*)

The label of choice is usually ^{125}I which gives a very high signal:noise ratio. The labeled antigen or antibody can be detected by direct counting in a gamma counter or by autoradiography with subsequent visual inspection or densitometry of the film. Antibodies may also be labeled with tritium for use in situations where a low energy emitter is advantageous (e.g. precise localization of intracellular antigens using autoradiography) [4–7].

Problems: Reagent has a very limited shelf life due to decreasing signal because of radioactive decay (the half-life of ^{125}I is 59.6 days), and to radio-damage of the protein. Involves the use of radioactive material, requiring a designated 'hot' room for the labeling procedure.

Fluorochrome labeling (see *Protocol 4*)

Fluorescein isothiocyanate (FITC) is the label of choice for immunofluorescence because the coupling procedure is extremely easy, works with nearly all antibodies, and the fluorescence signal emitted is relatively strong. For two-color analysis, tetramethylrhodamine isothiocyanate (TRITC), Texas red (TR) or phycoerythrin (PE) are often used. For flow cytometry using two, three or four colors the choice of fluorochrome will be determined by the laser and optical filter systems available [8–11].

6. Miles, L.E.M. and Hales, C.N. (1986) *Nature*, **219**, 186–189.
7. Billington, D., Jayson, G.G. and Maltby, P.J. (1992) *Radioisotopes*. BIOS Scientific Publishers, Oxford.
8. Coons, A.H., Creech, H.J., Jones, R.N. and Berliner, E. (1942) *J. Immunol*. 45, 159–170.
9. Goding, J.W. (1976) *J. Immunol. Methods* **13**, 215–226.
10. Oi, V.T., Glazer, A.N. and Stryer, L. (1982) *J. Cell Biol*. **93**, 981–986.
11. The, T.H. and Feltkamp, T.E.W. (1970) *Immunology*, **18**, 875–881.
12. Bayer, E.A. and Wilchek, M. (1990) *Methods Enzymol*. **184**, 138–160.
13. Guesdon, J.-L., Ternynck, T. and Avrameas, S. (1979) *J. Histochem. Cytochem*. **27**, 1131–1139.
14. Kendall, C., Ionescu Matiu, I. and Dreesman, G.R. (1983) *J. Immunol. Methods* **56**, 329–339.
15. Galfrè, G. and Milstein, C. (1981) *Methods Enzymol*. **73**, 3–46.
16. Coligan, J.E., Gates, F.T., Kimball, E.S. and Maloy, W.L. (1983) *Methods Enzymol*. **91**, 413–434.
17. Cuello, A.C., Priestly, J.V. and Milstein, C. (1982) *Proc. Natl Acad. Sci. USA* **79**, 665–669.
18. Langone, J.J. (1982) *Adv. Immunol*. **32**, 157–252.

Problems: Requires fluorescence microscope or flow cytometer for detection.

Biotin labeling (see *Protocol 5*)

Biotinylated antibodies can be detected using streptavidin which can be conjugated to a variety of labels (e.g. enzymes, ^{125}I, fluorochromes). Many such conjugates are commercially available. The affinity of binding of streptavidin to biotin is extremely high; 10^{15}/M [12–14].

Problems: Biotinylation can occur in the antigen-binding site and lead to a reduction in, or even abolition of, antigen binding.

Biosynthetic labeling

Provides stable incorporation of a label (^{35}S-methionine, ^{3}H lysine, ^{3}H arginine, ^{3}H leucine or ^{3}H phenylalanine) without the need for a chemical coupling reaction which might damage the antibody [15–18].

Problems: Requires growth of the monoclonal antibody-producing cell line in medium which is deficient in the amino acid used for the label. The labeled molecule has low specific activity. Not applicable to polyclonal antibody reagents.

Choice of method

Enzyme labeling for immunoassays, fluorescent labeling with FITC for immunofluorescence.

Protocols provided

1. *Measuring antibody concentration by UV absorbance*
2. *Labeling with horseradish peroxidase*
3. *Labeling with ^{125}I*
4. *Labeling with fluorochrome*
5. *Labeling with biotin*

The choice of label will, to a large extent, be determined by the assay system to be employed. For immunofluorescence of cell- or tissue-associated antigens the label will be a fluorochrome. An alternative is to use an enzyme-labeled antibody for immunohistochemistry. For immunoassay the choice will usually be an enzyme for use in an ELISA system, although radioisotopes are still used in some instances where sensitive RIA systems are required. Use of radiochemicals requires compliance with national or state regulations controlling the use of such reagents. Appropriate shielding should be used (e.g. [125]I radiation starter pack RPN2062 from Amersham provides a comprehensive shielding and containment package for ^{125}I users). Used under the specified conditions in the quantities normally found in the laboratory, ^{125}I is not thought to present any greater hazard to health than many other commonly used reagents.

In addition to labeling the antibody itself, it is possible to use a labeled ligand for the antibody, and this is a common approach in the case of *Staphyloccocus* protein A and *Streptococcus* protein G [18]. Note, however, that only a single layer of the immunoassay can contain antibody able to bind the ligand and, conversely, that not all classes of antibodies bind these ligands (human IgG1, IgG2 and IgG4, mouse IgG2a, IgG2b and IgG3 bind protein A strongly, all four human IgG subclasses bind protein G strongly, but mouse IgG1 only shows moderate binding). Another, more versatile, alternative is to incorporate biotin molecules into the antibody (or antigen), which is then detected with labeled streptavidin. Most commonly 'long arm' biotin is used which includes a spacer molecule.

A very large number of secondary antibodies, as well as immunoglobulin-binding ligands such as protein A and protein G, are commercially available as enzyme (usually alkaline phosphatase, AP, or horseradish peroxidase, HRP) and fluorochrome (usually fluorescein isothiocyanate, FITC, tetramethylrhodamine, TRITC, phycoerythrin, PE, or Texas red, TR) conjugates. In cases where the desired antibody conjugates are not commercially available, labeling of antibodies in the laboratory is usually very straightforward using one of the relevant protocols given (*Protocols 2–5*).

Protocol 1. **Measuring antibody concentration by UV absorbance**

Reagents

Antibody sample
Phosphate-buffered saline (PBS) pH 7.4

Equipment

Cuvette, UV transparent (Quartz) (1 cm light path)
Pipettes (e.g. 0.5–10 μl and 200–1000 μl)
Pipette tips
Test tubes (e.g. 55 × 11 mm, round bottom)
UV spectrophotometer

Technique

1. Fill a thoroughly clean cuvette with buffer. ①
2. Set the spectrophotometer to 280 nm and adjust the reading to zero using buffer alone.
3. Dilute purified antibody 1 in 100 in buffer. ②
4. Measure the absorbance of the diluted antibody. ③
5. Calculate the antibody concentration. ④

Notes

① If using a spectrophotometer equipped with a flow cell, wash through with distilled water and then load buffer into the flow cell.

② The antibody should be relatively pure otherwise contaminating proteins will influence the absorbance. Proteins precipitated from serum with 40% ammonium sulfate consist mostly of immunoglobulins and therefore the antibody concentration in such preparations can be roughly estimated using this technique.

③ If the reading is too high (over) make a higher dilution of antibody, e.g. 1 in 1000. If the reading is very low (<0.1) a more accurate value can be obtained by making a lower dilution of antibody, e.g. 1 in 20.

④ For IgG the concentration in mg/ml = A_{280} (the absorbance reading at 280 nm) × 0.70 × the dilution of antibody measured. For IgM multiply the absorbance reading by 0.84 and for IgA by 0.94.

Protocol 1. Measuring antibody concentration

Protocol 2. Labeling with horseradish peroxidase

Reagents

Antibody
Carbonate–bicarbonate buffer, pH 9.5
Horseradish peroxidase (HRP)
Phosphate-buffered saline (PBS) pH 7.4
1 mM Sodium acetate, pH 4.0
4 mg/ml Sodium borohydride ⚠, in double-distilled water
0.1 M Sodium periodate ⚠ in 10 mM sodium phosphate saline pH 7.0

Equipment

Beakers (1 liter)
Dialysis tubing, cellulose membrane
Magnetic stirrer
Pipettes (40–200 μl and 200–1000 μl)
Pipette tips
Test tubes (e.g. 55 × 11 mm, round bottom)

Technique

1 Dissolve 4 mg of HRP in 1 ml double-distilled water.

2 Add 240 µl of 0.1 M sodium periodate in 10 mM sodium phosphate saline pH 7.0. ①

3 Leave for 20 min at RT.

4 Dialyze against 1 mM sodium acetate pH 4.0 for 24 h with several changes of buffer.

5 Separately but concurrently dialyze 400 µl of 10 mg/ml purified antibody against carbonate–bicarbonate buffer pH 9.5 for 24 h with several changes of buffer.

6 Add dialyzed HRP to the dialyzed antibody.

Notes

① Prepared fresh each time.

② Conjugated antibodies should be stored at 4°C in the presence of 0.1% sodium azide. ⚠

7 Leave at RT for 2 h.

8 Add 100 µl of 4 mg/ml sodium borohydride in double-distilled water.

9 Incubate at 4°C for 2 h.

10 Dialyze against PBS pH 7.4 for 24 h with several changes of buffer. [1]

11 Titrate the antibody in the system to be used in order to determine the optimal dilution for use. ②

Pause point

[1] Can leave dialyzing for 3–4 days in PBS containing 0.1% sodium azide.

Protocol 2. Labeling with horseradish peroxidase

Protocol 3. Labeling with ^{125}I

NB This procedure must not be carried out until appropriate training has been received in the safe use of volatile radioactive iodine.

Reagents

Antibody

10 mg/ml Bovine serum albumin (BSA) in PBS with 0.1% sodium azide ⚠

Chloramine-T ⚠

Phosphate-buffered saline (PBS) pH 7.4

0.5 M Sodium phosphate buffer pH 7.4

Sodium (^{125}I) iodide (carrier free, 3.7 GBq/ml, 100 mCi/ml) ⚠

Equipment

Microcentrifuge

Microcentrifuge tubes

PD-10 column (pre-packed with Sephadex G-25) (Pharmacia)

Pipettes (e.g. 0.5–10 μl and 10–20 ml)

Pipette tips, 200–1000 μl

Radiation protection shield (e.g. 12 mm lead-impregnated acrylic)

Scintillation probe monitor

Technique

1 Pass 20 ml PBS, then 10 ml of 10 mg/ml BSA in PBS, then a further 20 ml PBS through a PD-10 column. ①

2 Put 10 µl of 0.5 M sodium phosphate buffer pH 7.4 into a microcentrifuge tube.

3 Add 10 µl of 1 mg/ml antibody in PBS and place tube behind appropriate shielding (e.g. ^{125}I radiation starter pack, Amersham International) in a ventilated enclosure in a designated radio-activity room. ②

4 Add 5 µl (18.5 MBq, 0.5 mCi) of Na ^{125}I.

Notes

① Keep column outlet capped after this equilibration step in order to prevent column drying out.

② After this step disposable latex medical gloves should be worn (ideally two pairs so that the top glove can be removed should it become contaminated). Place the microcentrifuge tube behind appropriate lead and/or lead-impregnated acrylic shielding (e.g. Scotlab, Amersham, etc). Monitor work station and yourself before and after each procedure.

③ The first peak contains the iodinated antibody, the second peak unincorporated Na ^{125}I. Discard all waste radioactive

5 Add 10 μl of 5 mg/ml chloramine-T in 0.5 M sodium phosphate buffer pH 7.4.

6 Mix with the tip of a pipette for 60 sec.

7 Pipette the contents of the iodination tube on to the top of the PD-10 column.

8 Elute the column with 10 ml PBS containing 10 mg/ml BSA, 0.1% sodium azide and collect 300 μl fractions into microcentrifuge tubes.

9 Assess radioactivity in each tube with a scintillation probe monitor and pool the tubes containing the first radioactive peak. ③

materials in strict accordance with local regulations. Radiolabeled antibodies should be stored in appropriate lead or lead-impregnated acrylic containers (e.g. ^{125}I safe storage box, Amersham International) at 4°C in the presence of 0.1% sodium azide.

Protocol 4. Labeling with fluorochrome

Reagents

Antibody
Carbonate–bicarbonate buffer pH 9.5
Dimethylsulfoxide (DMSO, anhydrous) ⚠
Fluorescein isothiocyanate (FITC) ⚠ (or tetramethylrhodamine
  (TRITC) ⚠ or Texas red (TR) ⚠) (NB Store in dessicator)
Phosphate-buffered saline (PBS) pH 7.4

Equipment

Beaker (1 liter)
Cuvette, UV transparent (Quartz) (1 cm light path)
Dialysis tubing, cellulose membrane
Magnetic stirrer
PD-10 column (pre-packed with Sephadex G-25) (Pharmacia)
Pipettes (e.g. 0.5–10 μl, 40–200 μl and 1–10 ml)
Pipette tips
Test tubes (e.g. 55 × 11 mm, round bottom)
UV spectrophotometer

Technique

1 Dialyze purified antibody against three changes of 500 ml of carbonate-bicarbonate buffer pH 9.5 at 4°C. ①

2 Remove the antibody from the dialysis tubing and measure the optical density (OD). ②

3 Calculate the amount of fluorochrome required at 10 µg/mg of antibody and dissolve FITC or TRITC in DMSO at 5 mg/ml. ③

4 Add 2 µl of FITC or TRITC to the antibody for each mg to be labeled. ④

Notes

① 6–8 h per buffer change. Buffer for TR is 0.025 M borate buffer pH 9.0.

② See *Protocol 1*.

③ Or use TR in cold acetonitrile ⚠ (anhydrous) at 1 mg/ml.

④ Or use 10 μl TR for each mg of antibody to be labeled.

⑤ Leave on melting ice for TR.

⑥ The conjugated antibody will be clearly visible on the column and will pass through much quicker than the lower molecular weight unincorporated fluorochrome.

5 Leave in the dark for 2 h at RT. ⑤

6 Pipette the labeled antibody on to the top of a PD-10 column.

7 Elute the column with 10 ml of PBS and collect the first peak of fluorescent material. ⑥ [1]

8 Measure the UV absorbance at 495 nm and 280 nm for FITC or at 550 nm and 280 nm for TRITC. ⑦

9 Titrate the antibody in the system to be used in order to determine the optimal dilution for use.

⑦ For FITC the ratio 495 nm:280 nm should be between 0.3 and 1.0, for TRITC 550 nm:280 nm should be between 0.2 and 0.3, and for TR 596 nm:280 nm should be between 0.7 and 0.9. If the ratios are outside these ranges, repeat the labeling procedure using lower or higher amounts of fluorochrome.

Pause point

[1] Conjugated antibodies should be stored at 4°C in the presence of 0.1% sodium azide. ⚠

Protocol 4. Labeling with fluorochrome

Protocol 5. Labeling with biotin

Reagents

Antibody
Bicarbonate–saline buffer: 0.1 M NaHCO$_3$ 0.1 M NaCl pH 7.4
Dimethylsulfoxide (DMSO) ⚠
Long arm biotin (e.g. biotinamidocaproate-N-hydroxysulfosuccinimide
  ester (BAC-SulfoNHS; Sigma))
Phosphate-buffered saline (PBS) pH 7.4
0.15 M NaCl

Equipment

Beaker (1 liter)
Cuvette, UV transparent (Quartz) (1 cm light path)
Dialysis tubing, cellulose membrane
Magnetic stirrer
Pipettes (e.g. 0.5–10 μl, 40–200 μl and 200–1000 μl)
Pipette tips
Test tubes (e.g. 55 × 11 mm, round bottom)
UV spectrophotometer

Technique

1 Dialyze purified antibody against three changes of 500 ml buffer. ①

2 Remove the antibody from the dialysis tubing and measure optical density (OD). ②

3 Calculate the amount of biotin required at 100 µg/mg of antibody. Dissolve the required amount of biotin in anhydrous DMSO at 6.8 mg/ml immediately prior to use. ③

4 Mix the biotin solution with the amount of antibody to be labeled and leave for 2 h at RT.

5 Remove unbound biotin by dialysis once in 0.15 M NaCl and then

Notes

① Leave on a magnetic stirrer for 6–8 h at 4°C for each change of buffer.

② See *Protocol 1*.

③ Biotinylation may interfere with antigen binding or other functional properties of the antibody. The risk can be reduced by using long arm biotin which contains a spacer between the protein-binding and streptavidin-binding sites.

④ Conjugated antibodies should be stored at 4°C in the presence of 0.1% sodium azide.

in two changes of PBS. ① 1

6 Remove biotinylated antibody from the dialysis tubing. ④

7 Titrate the antibody in the system to be used in order to determine the optimal dilution for use.

Pause points

1 Can leave dialyzing for 3–4 days in PBS containing 0.1% sodium azide. ⚠

III DETECTION AND QUANTIFICATION OF SOLUBLE ANTIGEN OR ANTIBODY

There are a number of immunological systems available which can be used to detect antibodies or antigens [1–6]. These assays rely either on the labeling of one of the reactants, on the formation of precipitating immune complexes, or on the measurement of an effector function of the antibody such as agglutination or complement fixation. The ability to make these assays quantitative depends upon the construction of a standard curve based on readings obtained using dilutions made from a known amount of the reactant; the amount of antigen in the unknown samples can then be read off from the curve.

Methods available

Enzyme-linked immunosorbent assay (ELISA) (see *Protocols 6–9*)
The assay of choice where soluble antigen is available. Relatively straightforward and able to handle a large number of samples. The antibody isotype can be determined using class/subclass-specific secondary antibodies [7–10].
Problems: Very few, but ensure adequate controls are included each time to exclude spurious cross-reactions, etc. May occasionally not be as accurate for quantification as some radioimmunoassays due to the limitations of the enzyme kinetics, although various amplification procedures can improve the sensitivity of ELISA.

Radioimmunoassay (RIA) (see *Protocol 10*)
Straightforward assay where soluble antigen is available and a radioactive detection system is preferred. May occasionally be more sensitive than a conventional ELISA. Ability to handle a large number of samples [11–15].
Problems: Involves the use of radioisotopes. A major disadvantage is the

References

1. Gosling, J.P. and Basso, L.V. (eds) (1994) *Immunoassay: Laboratory Analysis and Clinical Applications.* Butterworth-Heinemann, Boston.
2. Price, C.P. and Newman, D.J. (eds) (1991) *Principles and Practice of Immunoassay.* Stockton Press, New York.
3. Wild, D. (ed.) (1994) *The Immunoassay Handbook.* Stockton Press, New York.
4. Ekins, R.P. and Chu, F. (1994) *Trends Biotech.* **12**, 89–94.
5. Tijssen, P. (1985) *Practice and Theory of Immunoassay.* Elsevier, Amsterdam.
6. Yalow, R.S. and Berson, S.A. (1959) *Nature* **184**, 1648–1649.
7. Kemeny, D.M. and Challacombe, S.J. (eds) (1988) *ELISA and Other Solid Phase Immunoassays.* John Wiley and Sons, Chichester.
8. Engvall, E. and Perlmann, P. (1971) *Immunochemistry* **8**, 871–879.
9. Tijssen, P. and Adam, A. (1991) *Curr. Opin. Immunol.* **3**,

limited shelf life of the reagents due to the relatively short half-life of ^{125}I (59.6 days) and the potential for radioactive damage to the protein.

Immunoprecipitation in gels (see *Protocols 11–15*)

A number of different gel-based assays are available which rely either on the diffusion of one (single radial immunodiffusion) or both (double immunodiffusion) reactants, electrophoretic separation of the antigen followed by diffusion of the antibody (immunoelectrophoresis), or the electrophoretic migration of antigen and antibody towards each other (crossed (two-dimensional) electrophoresis). These techniques are very straightforward, particularly those not involving electrophoresis [16–20].

Problems: Not as sensitive as ELISA or RIA. Tedious and cumbersome if large numbers of samples are to be measured. For single radial immunodiffusion ensure that the gel has cooled sufficiently, but has not begun to set, before adding the antigen or antibody.

Nephelometry

As a method for quantification, immunonephelometry can be employed to measure light scattering by immune complexes. This is a sensitive and rapid technique that uses very small sample sizes (1–10 μl) [21–23].

Problems: Requires special equipment (laser nephelometer) not commonly present in most laboratories. Care is required in interpretation of the results as misleading readings may be obtained in antigen or antibody excess.

233–237.

10. Nilsson, B. (1990) *Curr. Opin. Immunol.* **2**, 898–904.
11. Catt, K.J. and Tregear, G. (1967) *Science* **158**, 1570–1572.
12. Vunakis, H.V. (1980) Radioimmunoassays: an overview. *Methods Enzymol.* **70**, 201–209.
13. Ekins, R. (1990) *Endocr. Rev.* **11**, 5–46.
14. de Medeiros, S.F, Amato, F., Matthews, C.D. and Norman, R.J. (1992) *J. Endocrinol.* **135**, 161–174.
15. Chard, T. (1990) *Radioimmunoassay and Related Techniques*, 4th Edn. Elsevier Science Publishers, Amsterdam.
16. Ouchterlony, Ö. and Nilsson, L.-A. (1986) in *Handbook of Experimental Immunology* (D.M Weir, L.A. Herzenberg, C. Blackwell and L.A. Herzenberg, eds), Vol 1. pp. 32.1–32.50. Blackwell Scientific Publications, Oxford.
17. Vaerman, J.-P. (1981) *Methods Enzymol.* **73**, 291–305.
18. Oudin, J. (1980) *Methods Enzymol.* **70**, 166–198.
19. Dunbar, B.S. (1988) *Two-dimensional Electrophoresis and Immunological Techniques*. Plenum Press, New York.
20. Heegaard, P.M.H. and Bøg-Hansen, T.C. (1986) in *Gel Electrophoresis of Proteins*. (M.J. Dunn, ed.), pp. 262–311.Wright, Bristol.
21. Nilsson, L.-A. (1992) in *Encyclopedia of Immunology* (I.M. Roitt and P.J. Delves, eds), pp. 1143–1144. Academic Press, London.
22. Höffken, K. and Schmidt, C.G. (1981) *Methods Enzymol.* **74**, 628–644.
23. Whicher, J.T., Price, C.P. and Spencer, K. (1983) *Crit. Rev. Clin. Lab. Sci.* **18**, 213–260.

Agglutination (see *Protocols 16* and *17*)

Very straightforward and can be fairly sensitive [24–27].

Problems: The antigen must first be coupled to erythrocytes or inert particles such as latex. Some polyclonal sera may contain antibodies capable of agglutinating erythrocytes.

Complement-fixation test

A sensitive assay that measures a biologically important function of the antibody molecule, i.e. the ability to activate complement [28–30].

Problems: Only measures those classes of antibody which are able to fix complement (IgM, IgG1, IgG3 (and IgG2 and IgA weakly) in man; IgM, IgG2a, IgG2b and IgG3 in mouse, IgG2a, IgG2b, IgG2c and IgM in rat). It is also a comparatively complex assay.

Choice of method

ELISA is the most straightforward broadly applicable method, either coating purified antigen on to the plate or using a capture antibody on the plate to first 'pull out' the antigen of interest from a mixture of antigens.

24. Adler, F.L. and Adler, L.T. (1980) *Methods Enzymol.* **70**, 455–466.
25. Poston, R.N. (1974) *J. Immunol. Methods* **5**, 91–96.
26. Maehara, T., Eda, Y., Mitani, K. and Matsuzawa, S. (1990) *Biomaterials* **11**, 122–126.
27. Wilson, K.M., Gerometta, M., Rylatt, D.B. *et al.* (1991) *J. Immunol. Methods* **138**, 111–119.
28. Borsos, T. (1992) in *Encyclopedia of Immunology* (I.M. Roitt and P.J. Delves, eds), pp. 381–382. Academic Press, London.
29. Swack, N.S., Gahan, T.F. and Hausler, W.J. Jr (1992) *Infect. Agents-Dis.* **1**, 219–224.
30. Artsob, H. and Huibner, S. (1990) *J. Clin. Microbiol.* **28**, 637–638.

Protocols provided

6. *Indirect ELISA*
7. *Sandwich ELISA*
8. *Competition ELISA for antigen*
9. *Inhibition ELISA for monoclonal antibody mapping*
10. *Fluid phase RIA*
11. *Pre-coating glass slides with agarose*
12. *Double immunodiffusion*
13. *Single radial immunodiffusion*
14. *Immunoelectrophoresis*
15. *Crossed (two-dimensional) electrophoresis*
16. *Conjugation of antigen to erythrocytes*
17. *Immunoagglutination*

ELISA *(Protocols 6–9)*

For most antigens, Immulon II ELISA plates (Dynatech) should produce satisfactory results. Where there is a necessity for a very high degree of sensitivity and inter-plate reproducibility then the more expensive higher grades of plate may prove useful. Coating of ELISA plates overnight at 4°C is convenient but times can be shortened to 1–4 h, in which case the plates should be incubated at 37°C. Plates are usually coated with 3–5 μg/ml of antigen but higher concentrations (e.g. 10 μg/μl) can be tried, as can other coating buffers (e.g. bicarbonate–carbonate buffer pH 9.6 in place of PBS pH 7.4), should the assay prove to have low sensitivity. If antigen is limited, the coating volume can be reduced to 50 μl. In the case of particularly precious antigens, the coating solution can be carefully removed from the wells (e.g. using a multichannel pipette) and re-used, as the binding capacity of the plastic is usually less than 3 μg/ml. A pilot experiment should be carried out to ascertain if this can be done without a significant loss of sensitivity. Ideally, carry out subsequent coatings immediately. Otherwise, store the coating solution at 4°C with 0.1% sodium azide in a siliconized glass container. If high backgrounds are encountered in an ELISA, different blocking agents can be tried, e.g. 1% BSA, 1% fetal calf serum (FCS) or 0.05% Tween 20. Blocking times can usually be reduced, for example to 20 min at 37°C.

Positive and negative controls for the ELISA should be included on every plate and all assay points done in duplicate, including the controls. A positive control would be an antibody known to bind to the antigen, a negative control would be one that is known not to bind to the antigen. The dilution of test antibodies will depend on the aim of the experiment, for example if testing antisera for specificity to a given antigen, dilutions of 1:10, 1:100 and 1:1000 might be appropriate. Increased incubation times, for example overnight, may increase the binding. It is important that once a set of conditions (time, temperature, washes, reagent concentrations) are established, that they are adhered to for every experiment in a given study. Occasionally, a fluid phase radioimmunoassay may provide sensitivity greater than that normally achieved using ELISA techniques.

To wash ELISA plates, hold the plate upright over the sink and then very quickly invert the plate with a throwing action (but do not let go!) so that the contents of the wells are rapidly expelled. Quickly fill the wells with buffer from a squirt bottle. After three cycles of wash/discard, the plate should be banged upside down on to some folded paper towel to remove any remaining liquid. Quickly proceed

Soluble antigen or antibody

to the next step without allowing the plate to dry out. ELISA plate washing machines of various degrees of sophistication are also available. Keep plates wrapped in Clingfilm (polyvinylchloride film) at all incubation steps. (See *Protocols 6–9*.)

Secondary (labeled) antibodies can be either monoclonal or polyclonal, raised in any species that will not cause problems of cross-reactivity, and can be against different heavy or light chain isotypes if desired. The protocols provided are based on using horseradish peroxidase- or alkaline phosphatase-labeled antibodies, although other enzymes, for example β-galactosidase, can be used in the very rare instances where neither of the aforementioned enzymes proves suitable. It is also possible to use other labeled immunoglobulin-binding ligands such as protein G or protein A. The enzyme reaction is normally stopped when the positive control has developed a strong color. Following addition of the substrate, the plates should be incubated in the dark, except when checking the progress of the enzyme reaction. Do not let the plate overdevelop as this will prevent quantitative measurements being achieved. The enzyme reactions are normally stopped by changing the pH. A variety of ELISA plate readers are available. If only determining positivity, for example of hybridoma supernatants, an ELISA plate reader is unnecessary as the plates can be visually inspected for wells in which a color reaction has occurred.

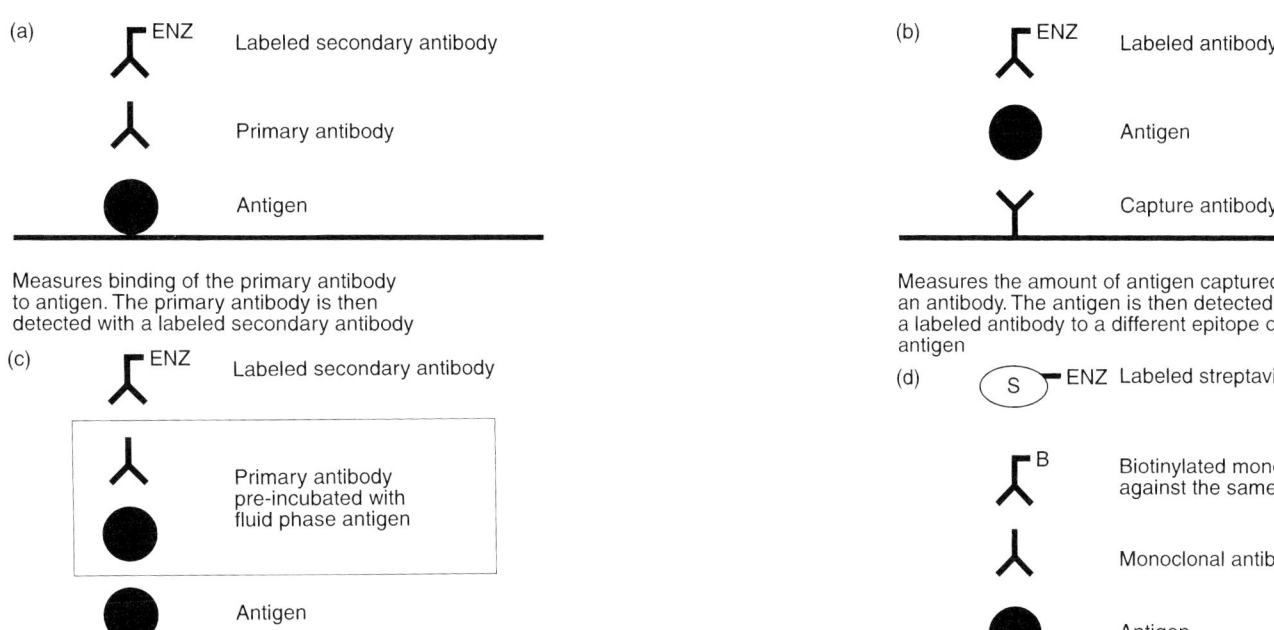

(a) ENZ — Labeled secondary antibody

Primary antibody

Antigen

Measures binding of the primary antibody to antigen. The primary antibody is then detected with a labeled secondary antibody

(b) ENZ — Labeled antibody

Antigen

Capture antibody

Measures the amount of antigen captured by an antibody. The antigen is then detected using a labeled antibody to a different epitope on the antigen

(c) ENZ — Labeled secondary antibody

Primary antibody pre-incubated with fluid phase antigen

Antigen

Measures amount of antigen by the ability of fluid phase antigen to competitively inhibit the binding of an antibody to the solid phase antigen

(d) S — ENZ Labeled streptavidin

B — Biotinylated monoclonal antibody against the same antigen

Monoclonal antibody

Antigen

Measures ability of one antibody to inhibit antigen binding of the other antibody

Figure 2. Protocols for ELISAs with the following configurations are provided: (a) indirect ELISA; (b) sandwich ELISA (c) competition ELISA for antigen; (d) inhibition ELISA for monoclonal antibody mapping.

31

Soluble antigen or antibody

Protocol 6. **Indirect ELISA**

Reagents

Primary antibody (test samples, positive and negative controls)
Antigen
4% Dried skimmed milk powder (e.g. Marvel) in PBS (blocking agent)
4% Dried skimmed milk powder (e.g. Marvel) plus 0.05% Tween 20 in PBS (ELISA buffer)
Horseradish peroxidase (HRP) (or alkaline phosphatase (AP))-labeled anti-immunoglobulin (against primary antibody)
Phosphate-buffered saline (PBS) pH 7.4
Substrate: Tetramethylbenzidine (TMB) ⚠ for HRP, *p*-nitrophenyl phosphate (pNPP) ⚠ for AP (see ④).
Sulfuric acid, 12% ⚠
Tween 20, 0.05% in PBS (PBS-T)

Equipment

Absorbent paper towel
Clingfilm (polyvinylchloride film)
ELISA plates (e.g. Immulon II, Dynatech)
ELISA plate reader
Pipettes (single and multi-channel) (e.g. 0.5–10 μl and 40–200 μl)
Pipette tips
Squirt bottle

Technique

1 Place 100 µl/well of antigen at 3 µg/ml in PBS into the required number of wells of an ELISA plate. Keep plate upright and wrap in Clingfilm. Leave overnight at 4°C. ①

2 Wash the plate three times with PBS.

3 Add 200 µl/well of 4% milk powder in PBS and leave for 1 h at RT. ②

4 Wash the plate three times with PBS-T.

Notes

See pp. 29–31.

① Duplicate wells for all samples including positive (antibody known to bind the antigen) and negative (antibody known not to bind the antigen) controls.

② Alternatively can use AP-labeled antibody.

③ Once in PBS-T and twice in distilled water if using AP-labeled antibody.

5 Add 100 µl/well of primary antibodies diluted (e.g. 1 in 100) in ELISA buffer and leave for 2 h at RT. ①

6 Wash the plate three times with PBS-T.

7 Add 100 µl/well of a predetermined optimal concentration of HRP-labeled anti-Ig in ELISA buffer and leave for 2 h at RT. ②

8 Wash the plate three times with PBS-T. ③

9 Add 100 µl/well of TMB substrate and leave at RT in the dark. ④

10 Once sufficient color has developed in the positive wells add 50 µl/well of 12% sulfuric acid to stop the reaction. ⑤ ③

11 Measure the absorbance at 450 nm using an ELISA plate reader. ⑥

④ Dissolve 0.1 mg of TMB ⚠ in 100 µl DMSO ⚠. Add 9.9 ml of 0.1 M sodium acetate pH 6.0 and 3.3 µl of 30% hydrogen peroxide ⚠ immediately before use. For AP-labeled anti-immunoglobulin dissolve 10 mg of pNPP in 10 ml of 0.5 mM $MgCl_2$, 10 mM diethanolamine ⚠ pH 9.5.

⑤ Stop AP reaction with 3 M NaOH. ⚠

⑥ 405 nm for pNPP.

Pause points

1 Can be left tightly wrapped in Clingfilm for several days at 4°C if the PBS contains 0.1% sodium azide. ⚠

2 Can be left tightly wrapped in Clingfilm for several days at 4°C if the blocking agent contains 0.1% sodium azide.

3 The developed ELISA plates can be wrapped tightly in Clingfilm and stored in the dark at 4°C prior to reading.

Protocol 6. Indirect ELISA

Protocol 7. **Sandwich ELISA**

Reagents

Antigen
Capture antibody (monoclonal antibody specific for antigen of interest)
4% Dried skimmed milk powder (e.g. Marvel) in PBS (blocking agent)
4% Dried skimmed milk powder (e.g. Marvel) plus 0.05% Tween 20 in PBS (ELISA buffer)
Horseradish peroxidase (HRP) (or alkaline phosphatase (AP))-labeled detection antibody (specific for antigen of interest)
Phosphate-buffered saline (PBS) pH 7.4
Samples to be tested for presence of antigen
Substrate: Tetramethylbenzidine (TMB) ⚠ for HRP, p-nitrophenyl phosphate (pNPP) ⚠ for AP (see ④)
12% Sulfuric acid ⚠
0.05% Tween 20 in PBS (PBS-T)

Equipment

Absorbent paper towel
Clingfilm (polyvinylchloride film)
ELISA plates (e.g. Immulon II, Dynatech)
ELISA plate reader
Pipettes (single and multi-channel) (e.g. 0.5–10 μl and 40–200 μl)
Pipette tips
Squirt bottle

Technique

1 Place 100 µl/well of capture antibody at 3 µg/ml in PBS into the required number of wells of an ELISA plate. Keep plate upright and wrap in Clingfilm. Leave overnight at 4°C. [1]

2 Wash the plate three times with PBS.

3 Add 200 µl/well of 4% milk powder in PBS and leave for 1 h at RT. [2]

Notes

See pp. 29–31.

① Use duplicate wells for all samples including positive (antigen) and negative (irrelevant antigen) controls. If using assay for quantification, include a standard curve of known concentrations of purified antigen on each plate.

② Alternatively use a monoclonal antibody, which must be

4 Wash the plate three times with PBS-T.

5 Add 100 µl/well of test samples diluted (e.g. 1 in 100) in ELISA buffer and leave for 2 h at RT. ①

6 Wash the plate three times with PBS-T.

7 Add 100 µl/well of a predetermined optimal concentration of HRP- (or AP-) labeled antigen-specific polyclonal antibody in ELISA buffer and leave for 2 h at RT. ②

8 Wash the plate three times with PBS-T. ③

9 Add 100 µl/well TMB substrate and leave at RT in the dark. ④

10 Once sufficient color has developed in the positive wells add 50 µl/well of 12% sulfuric acid to stop the reaction. ⑤ ③

11 Measure absorbance at 450 nm using an ELISA plate reader. ⑥

directed against a different epitope region on the antigen to that recognized by the capture antibody.

③ Once in PBS-T and twice in distilled water if using an AP-labeled detection antibody.

④ Dissolve 0.1 mg of TMB⚠ in 100 µl DMSO ⚠. Add 9.9 ml of 0.1 M sodium acetate pH 6.0 and 3.3. µl of 30% hydrogen peroxide ⚠ immediately before use. For AP-labeled antibodies dissolve 10 mg of pNPP in 10 ml of 0.5 mM MgCl$_2$,10 mM diethanolamine ⚠ pH9.5.

⑤ Stop AP reaction with 50 µl/well of 3 M NaOH. ⚠

⑥ 405 nm for pNPP.

Pause points

1. Can be left tightly wrapped in Clingfilm for several days at 4°C if the PBS contains 0.1% sodium azide. ⚠

2. Can be left tightly wrapped in Clingfilm for several days at 4°C if the blocking agent contains 0.1% sodium azide. ⚠

3. The developed ELISA plates can be wrapped tightly in Clingfilm and stored in the dark at 4°C prior to reading.

Protocol 7. Sandwich ELISA

Protocol 8. **Competition ELISA for antigen**

Reagents

Antigen-specific primary antibody
Antigen (purified and test samples)
4% Dried skimmed milk powder (e.g. Marvel) in PBS (blocking agent)
4% Dried skimmed milk powder (e.g. Marvel) plus 0.05% Tween 20 in PBS (ELISA buffer)
Horseradish peroxidase (HRP)- (or alkaline phosphatase (AP))-labeled anti-immunoglobulin (against primary antibody)
Phosphate-buffered saline (PBS) pH 7.4
Substrate: Tetramethylbenzidine (TMB)⚠for HRP, p-nitrophenyl phosphate (pNPP)⚠ for AP (see ④).
12% Sulfuric acid ⚠
0.05% Tween 20 in PBS (PBS-T)

Equipment

Absorbent paper towel
Clingfilm (polyvinylchloride film)
ELISA plates (e.g. Immulon II, Dynatech)
ELISA plate reader
Pipettes (single and multi-channel) (e.g. 0.5–10 μl and 40–200 μl)
Pipette tips
Squirt bottle

Technique

1 Place 100 µl/well of antigen at 3 µg/ml in PBS into the required number of wells of an ELISA plate. Keep plate upright and wrap in Clingfilm. Leave overnight at 4°C.

2 At the same time, in blocked microtiter plates or microcentrifuge tubes, set up a dilution series of test antigen with a fixed amount of specific antibody in ELISA buffer. The final concentration of antibody should be ~80% of the saturating concentration in a binding curve (see *Figure 1,*

Notes

See pp. 29–31.

① If using the assay for quantification, include known amounts of inhibiting purified antigen so that a standard curve can be constructed.

② Alternatively use AP-labeled anti-Ig.

③ Once in PBS-T and twice in distilled water if using AP-conjugated reagent.

p.7). Leave overnight at 4°C. ①

3 Following overnight incubation, wash the coated ELISA plate (step 1) three times with PBS.

4 Add 200 µl/well of 4% milk powder in PBS to block the ELISA plate and leave for 1 h at RT.

5 Wash the plate three times with PBS-T.

6 Add 100 µl/well of the antibody which was incubated overnight with antigen (step 2) and leave on the ELISA plate for 2 h at RT.

7 Wash the plate three times with PBS-T.

8 Add 100 µl/well of a predetermined optimal concentration of HRP-labeled anti-Ig in ELISA buffer and leave for 2 h at RT. ②

9 Wash the plate three times with PBS-T. ③

10 Add 100 µl/well of TMB substrate and leave at RT in the dark. ④

11 Once sufficient color has developed in the positive wells add 50 µl/well of 12% sulfuric acid to stop the reaction. ⑤ [1]

12 Measure absorbance at 450 nm using an ELISA plate reader. ⑥

④ Dissolve 0.1 mg of TMB ⚠ in 100 µl DMSO ⚠. Add 9.9 ml of 0.1 M sodium acetate pH 6.0 and 3.3. µl of 30% hydrogen peroxide ⚠ immediately before use. For AP-labeled anti-immunoglobulin dissolve 10 mg of pNPP in 10 ml of 0.5 mM MgCl₂, 10 mM diethanolamine ⚠ pH 9.5.

⑤ Stop AP reaction with 3 M NaOH. ⚠

⑥ 405 nm for pNPP.

Pause point

[1] The developed ELISA plates can be wrapped tightly in Clingfilm and stored in the dark at 4°C prior to reading.

Protocol 8. Competition ELISA for antigen

Protocol 9. Inhibition ELISA for monoclonal antibody mapping

Reagents

Antigen

Biotinylated and unlabeled versions of MAbs to antigen of interest

4% Dried skimmed milk powder (e.g. Marvel) in PBS (blocking agent)

4% Dried skimmed milk powder (e.g. Marvel) in 0.05% Tween 20 in PBS (ELISA buffer)

Horseradish peroxidase (HRP)- (or alkaline phosphatase (AP))-labeled streptavidin

Phosphate-buffered saline (PBS) pH 7.4

Substrate: Tetramethylbenzidine (TMB) ⚠ for HRP, p-nitrophenyl phosphate (pNPP) ⚠ for AP (see ③)

12% Sulfuric acid ⚠

0.05% Tween 20 in PBS (PBS-T)

Equipment

Absorbent paper towel

Clingfilm (polyvinylchloride film)

ELISA plates (e.g. Immulon II, Dynatech)

ELISA plate reader

Pipettes (single and multi-channel) (e.g. 0.5–10 μl and 40–200 μl)

Pipette tips

Squirt bottle

Technique

1 Place 100 µl/well of antigen at 3 µg/ml in PBS into the required number of wells of an ELISA plate. Keep the plate upright and wrap in Clingfilm. Leave overnight at 4°C. ☐1

2 Wash the plate three times with PBS.

3 Add 200 µl/well of 4% milk powder in PBS and leave for 1 h at RT. ☐2

Notes

See pp. 29–31.

① The positive control would be the unlabeled form of this monoclonal antibody, and a negative control would be a monoclonal antibody known to bind to a different epitope on the same antigen or directed against an irrelevant antigen.

② Streptavidin binds with very high affinity to biotin.

③ Dissolve 0.1 mg of TMB ⚠ in 100 μl DMSO ⚠. Add 9.9 ml of 0.1 M sodium acetate pH 6.0 and 3.3 μl of 30% hydro-

4 Wash the plate three times with PBS-T.

5 Add 100 µl/well of a dilution series of the test monoclonal antibody diluted in ELISA buffer and leave for 2 h at RT.

6 Wash the plate three times with PBS-T.

7 Add 100 µl/well of a predetermined nonsaturating concentration of biotin-labeled monoclonal antibody in ELISA buffer and leave for 2 h at RT. ①

8 Wash the plate three times with PBS-T.

9 Add 100 µl/well of a predetermined optimal concentration of HRP-labeled strepavidin in ELISA buffer and leave for 2 h at RT. ②

10 Add 100 µl/well of TMB substrate. ③

11 Leave the plates in the dark at RT until color development in the positive wells and then add 50 µl/well of 12% sulfuric acid to stop the reaction. ④ ③

12 Measure absorbance at 450 nm using an ELISA plate reader. ⑤

gen peroxide ⚠ immediately before use. For AP-labeled streptavidin dissolve 10 mg of pNPP in 10 ml of 0.5 mM $MgCl_2$, 10 mM diethanolamine ⚠ pH 9.5.

④ Stop AP reaction with 3 M NaOH. ⚠

⑤ 405 nm for pNPP.

Pause points

[1] Plates can be left tightly wrapped in Clingfilm for several days at 4°C if the PBS contains 0.1% sodium azide. ⚠

[2] Plates can be left tightly wrapped in Clingfilm for several days at 4°C if the blocking agent contains 0.1% sodium azide.

[3] The developed ELISA plates can be wrapped tightly in Clingfilm and stored at 4°C prior to reading.

Protocol 9. Inhibition ELISA for monoclonal antibody mapping

RIA (*Protocol 10*)

Any of the ELISA-based assays described above can alternatively be carried out as RIAs by substituting iodinated antibody for the enzyme-labeled antibody. RIA can also be carried out in the fluid phase and an example of such an assay is given below. The nonlabeled antigen in the test sample competes with radiolabeled antigen for binding to antibody. The higher the concentration of nonlabeled antigen, the less radiolabeled antigen will bind. The amount of bound radiolabeled antigen is then measured following immunoprecipitation of antibody–antigen complexes in order to separate bound from free antigen. Although in the example below fixed *Staphylococcus aureus* is used as the precipitating agent, any reagent capable of precipitating the antibody can be substituted (e.g. protein A-coated agarose, a precipitating anti-immunoglobulin, etc.).

Reagents

Antibody

Antigen (purified and test samples)

Fixed *Staphylococcus aureus* Cowan 1 (SAC) (e.g. TACHISORB, Calbiochem)

^{125}I-labeled antigen ▽ (tracer) (e.g. ~74 TBq/mmol, 2000 Ci/mmol)

RIA buffer: 1% bovine serum albumin (BSA), 0.1% sodium azide ▽, 0.025% Tween 20 in PBS

Equipment

End-over-end mixer

Gamma-counter

^{125}I-scintillation probe monitor

Microcentrifuge

Microcentrifuge tubes

Pipettes (0.5–10 µl, 40–200 µl and 200–1000 µl)

Pipette tips

Radiation protection shield (e.g. 12 mm lead-impregnated acrylic)

Waste trap

Water bath or incubator, 37°C

Technique

1 Make a dilution series of the purified antigen in RIA buffer. ①

2 Incubate 100 μl of specific antibody, 100 μl of test samples (and the dilution series of purified antigen), and 50 μl of radiolabeled tracer antigen in microcentrifuge tubes at 37°C for 1 h. Include two or three dilutions (e.g. 1 in 10 and 1 in 100) for each test sample and carry out all assay points in duplicate. ②

3 Add 500 μl of SAC to each tube and mix. ③

4 Incubate for 20 min at 37°C on an end-over-end mixer.

5 Centrifuge at 10 000 g for 15 sec.

6 Wash pellet twice in 1 ml of RIA buffer by centrifugation at 10 000 g for 15 sec followed by removal of buffer after each centrifugation. ④ ☐1

7 Count precipitated pellets in a gamma-counter.

8 Draw a standard curve from the dilution series of purified antigen and use this to calculate the concentrations of the test samples.

Notes

① e.g. fourfold from 10 μg/ml.

② Rules for the handling and disposal of all radioactive material must be rigorously adhered to. Many antigens (e.g. hormones) are commercially available in radiolabeled form. If antigens need to be labeled (*Protocol 3*) this must be done in a designated radioactive suite for the safe handling of Na ^{125}I following expert training in the procedures involved. The amount of both tracer and of specific antibody must first be determined by constructing binding curves. The antibody will usually be used at somewhere between 1:1000 and 1:100 000. Only very small amounts of radiolabeled tracer antigen are required (≤ 20 000 cpm).

③ Use manufacturer's recommended concentration or determine empirically.

④ Wash buffer should be collected into a radioactivity waste trap (e.g. side arm flask).

Pause point

☐1 Pellets can be kept for a few days at RT before counting if necessary.

Immunoprecipitation in gels (*Protocols 11–15*)

The double immunodiffusion (Ouchterlony) technique (*Protocol 12*) is the simplest of the immunoprecipitation in gel techniques and relies on the diffusion of the reactants out of wells towards each other. Crossed (two-dimensional) electrophoresis (*Protocol 15*) is similar but uses electrophoresis to speed up the migration of the antibody and antigen towards each other, resulting in a precipitin band forming within one hour rather than overnight. It also requires less antigen and antibody because the electrophoresis drives the reactants towards each other, rather than them diffusing 360° from the well. In single radial immunodiffusion (*Protocol 13*) one of the reactants is incorporated into the gel itself and the other reactant diffuses out of a well to form a ring rather than a band of precipitation. Immunoelectrophoresis (*Protocol 14*) relies on the electrophoretic separation of an antigen mixture into its component parts prior to immunoprecipitation by antibody diffusing from a trough in the gel.

Pouring agarose on to glass slides requires a bit of practice and it is important to ensure an even thickness of gel. Use a spirit level to determine if the laboratory bench is level, and if not use either a purpose-made leveling tray or improvise using a glass plate and plasticine. Agarose solutions are prepared by heating in a microwave oven or on a stirring hotplate until all the agarose is dissolved. The agarose should be well above its setting temperature, the glass slide should be clean, and the agarose dispersed quickly so as to cover the entire slide. Pre-coating the slides with agarose (*Protocol 11*) greatly facilitates adhesion of the final agarose layer to the glass. The pre-coated slides can be stored at room temperature for several weeks until required.

After the final agarose layer has set on the glass slide, holes need to be cut in the gel so that the relevant antibody or antigen can be added. This is most easily achieved using a commercially available gel punch (e.g. from E-C Apparatus) but can also be carried out using the narrow end of a Pasteur pipette. The core of agarose is then removed and discarded; this is best done using a Pasteur pipette attached to a vacuum line, or alternatively pick it out with a needle. Commonly used well patterns are shown below (*Figures 3–6*) for the different techniques, together with the expected precipitation results. For immunoelectrophoresis it is also necessary to cut a trough in the agarose, using either a commercial cutter (e.g. from E–C Apparatus) or two appropriately spaced one-edged razor blades (e.g. separated by a thin piece of card and held together with adhesive tape). The gel should not be allowed to dry out and therefore should be kept in a humidified box made by placing a well-dampened tissue in a container such as a sandwich box. Make sure the lid is firmly replaced after placing slides in the box.

The bands of precipitation are most readily visualized by staining with Coomassie brilliant blue followed by destaining until the background stain has been washed out, leaving strongly stained bands of precipitation. Once dry, the gel can be kept for many years as a visual record of the experiment. Preservation is aided by covering the dried gel with adhesive tape.

Double immunodiffusion

Antibody is placed in the central well and test antigen in the outer wells. Two lines of precipitation which cross each other indicate that the antiserum recognizes two unrelated antigens. If the lines were to merge into one another this would indicate that the two antigens are recognized similarly by the antiserum (although they are not necessarily identical). If they merge but one of the lines also continues (to give a 'spur') there is partial identity between the antigens in terms of recognition by the antiserum (see *Figure 3*).

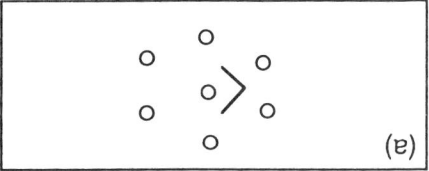 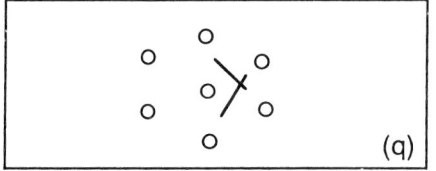 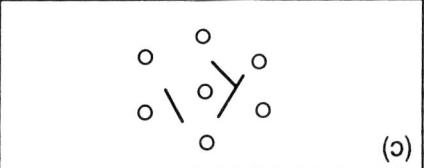

Figure 3. Double immunodiffusion. (a) Pattern shows identical recognition of antigen in two adjacent wells, but no reactivity with antigen in the remaining four wells. The two precipitin bands fuse at the point of contact. (b) Pattern shows unrelated recognition of antigen in two adjacent wells and no reactivity with antigen in the remaining four wells. The two precipitin bands cross each other without fusing. (c) Indicates partial identity of the recognition of antigen in two adjacent wells. One of the two precipitin bands extends out from the point of fusion to form a spur. There is also reactivity with antigen in one of the other wells.

Single radial immunodiffusion

The radius of the precipitin ring is related to the amount of specific antibody or antigen in the well. The assay can therefore be made quantitative by testing a range of known concentrations and constructing a standard curve of concentration versus radius. The concentration of the unknown test samples can then be ascertained by measuring the radius of the ring of precipitation and reading the concentration from the standard curve (see *Figure 4*).

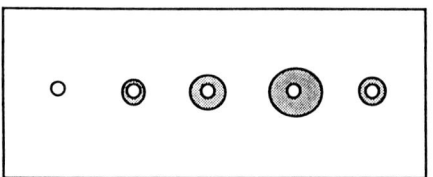

Figure 4. Single radial immunodiffusion. In this example, an antiserum in the gel does not detect any antigen in the left hand well. There are increasing amounts of antigen recognized in the next three wells. The right hand well contains a roughly similar amount of antigen to that found in the second well from the left.

Immunoelectrophoresis
Antigen is first subjected to electrophoretic separation, then the central trough is filled with antiserum. The relative positions of the different bands of precipitation formed are interpreted by comparison with standard patterns obtained with known antigens (see *Figure 5*).

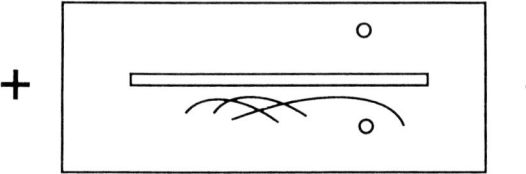

Figure 5. Immunoelectrophoresis. Antiserum produces multiple bands of precipitation with the antigens in the lower well, but does not recognize any components of the antigens in the upper well.

Crossed (two-dimensional) electrophoresis

Antibody and antigen are electrophoresed towards each other (see *Figure 6*).

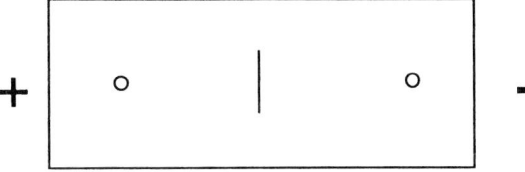

Figure 6. Crossed (two-dimensional) electrophoresis. The band of precipitation indicates that the antibody recognizes the antigen.

Protocol 11. Pre-coating glass slides with agarose

Reagents

Agarose (EEO 0.09–0.13)
Distilled water

Equipment

Beaker (e.g. 100 ml)
Glass slides (26 × 76 mm)
Incubator (37°C)
Leveling tray
Microwave or stirring hotplate
Pipette (5 ml)
Spirit level

Technique

1 Dissolve agarose at 1 mg/ml in distilled water by heating in a microwave oven or on a stirring hot plate.

2 Pipette 5 ml of molten agarose on to a clean glass slide. ①

3 Once the agarose has set (approximately 5–10 min) incubate the slide at 37°C until dry.

Notes

① Placed on a level bench or leveling tray.

Protocol 12. Double immunodiffusion

Reagents

Agarose (EEO 0.09–0.13)
Antibody solution
Antigen solution
0.05% (v/v) Coomassie brilliant blue R, in 50% methanol ⚠ , 10% glacial acetic acid ⚠
Distilled water
7% Glacial acetic acid ⚠, in 5% methanol ⚠
Phosphate-buffered saline (PBS) pH 7.4

Equipment

Absorbent paper towel
Beaker (e.g. 100 ml)
3MM chromatography paper (Whatman)
Gel punch
Leveling tray
Microwave or stirring hotplate
Orbital shaker
Pipettes (e.g. 0.5–10 μl and 5 ml)
Pipette tips
Pre-coated glass slides (*Protocol 11*)
Sandwich box
Spirit level

Technique

1 Dissolve agarose at 10 mg/ml in PBS by heating in a microwave oven or on a stirring hotplate.

2 Pipette 5 ml of molten agarose on to a pre-coated glass slide on a level surface and allow to set. ☐1

3 Cut holes in the agarose. ①

4 Fill each well with 10 µl of antigen or antibody solution. ②

Notes

① See *Figure 3*, p. 43.

② For example, specific antibody is placed in the center well and different antigen solutions including one known to contain the antigen of interest (i.e. a positive control) are placed in the outer wells. Some gel punches produce smaller wells (e.g. 5 μl).

③ If required, the gel can be re-dried by placing between sheets of 3MM paper with a weight on top.

5 Leave overnight at RT in a humidified box. ☐2

6 Wash the gel extensively by very gentle agitation in six changes of distilled water over a period of 24 h.

7 Dry the gel overnight at RT by covering with two sheets of Whatman 3MM paper.

8 Peel off the 3MM paper and stain the gel by submerging in Coomassie brilliant blue staining solution for 5 min.

9 Destain by very gentle agitation in 5% methanol, 7% glacial acetic acid.

10 Examine the gel for bands of precipitation. ③

Pause points

☐1 Can be kept in a humidified box at 4°C for 2–3 days if necessary.

☐2 Can be kept in a humidified box at 4°C for 2–3 days if necessary.

Protocol 13. Single radial immunodiffusion

Reagents

Agarose (EEO 0.09–0.13)
Antibody solution
Antigen solution
0.05% (v/v) Coomassie brilliant blue R, in 50% methanol ⚠, 10% glacial acetic acid ⚠
Distilled water
7% Glacial acetic acid ⚠, in 5% methanol ⚠
Phosphate-buffered saline (PBS) pH 7.4

Equipment

Absorbent paper towel
Beaker (e.g. 100 ml)
3MM chromatography paper (Whatman)
Gel punch
Leveling tray
Microwave or stirring hotplate
Orbital shaker
Pipettes (e.g. 0.5–10 μl and 5 ml)
Pipette tips
Pre-coated glass slides (*Protocol 11*)
Sandwich box
Spirit level
Thermometer

Technique

1 Dissolve agarose at 10 mg/ml in PBS by heating in a microwave oven or on a stirring hotplate.

2 When the agarose has cooled to 56°C add antigen to give a final antigen concentration of 1 mg/ml. ①

Notes

① This is most easily achieved by allowing the agarose to cool in a 56°C water bath.

② See *Figure 4* p. 44.

③ If a quantitative analysis is being undertaken, several measurements should be carried out using a range of known anti-

3 Pipette 5 ml of the antigen-containing molten agarose on to a pre-coated glass slide on a level surface and allow to set. [1]

4 Cut a row of small holes in the agarose. ②

5 Fill the wells with 10 µl of antibody. ③

6 Leave overnight at RT in a humidified box. [2]

7 Wash the gel extensively by very gentle agitation in six changes of distilled water over a period of 24 h.

8 Dry the gel overnight at RT by covering with two sheets of Whatman 3MM paper.

9 Peel off the 3MM paper and stain the gel by submerging in Coomassie brilliant blue staining solution for 5 min.

10 Destain by very gentle agitation in 5% methanol, 7% glacial acetic acid.

11 Measure the radius of the precipitin rings and calculate the concentration of the unknown samples based upon the graph derived from the known samples.

body concentrations. A calibration line can then be plotted (radius of precipitation versus antibody concentration) and the unknown antibody concentration estimated. The assay is often used to measure antigen in which case the antibody is incorporated in to the agarose (Step 2) and antigen placed in the wells. Some gel punches produce smaller wells (e.g. 5 µl).

Pause points

[1] Can be kept in a humidified box at 4°C for 2–3 days if necessary.

[2] Can be kept in a humidified box at 4°C for 2–3 days if necessary.

Protocol 13. Single radial immunodiffusion

Protocol 14. Immunoelectrophoresis

Reagents

Agarose (EEO 0.09–0.13)
Antibody solution
Antigen solution
0.0005% Bromophenol blue ⚠
0.05% (v/v) Coomassie brilliant blue R, in 50% methanol ⚠, 10%
   glacial acetic acid ⚠
Distilled water
7% Glacial acetic acid, in 5% methanol ⚠
Phosphate-buffered saline (PBS) pH 7.4
Tris-barbital buffer pH 8.6 ⚠

Equipment

Absorbent paper towel
Beaker (e.g. 100 ml)
3MM chromatography paper (Whatman)
Electrophoresis tank (e.g. Multiphor II, Pharmacia)
Gel punch
Leveling tray
Microwave or stirring hotplate
Orbital shaker
Pipettes (e.g. 0.5–10 μl, 40–200 μl and 5ml)
Pipette tips
Power pack
Pre-coated glass slides (*Protocol 11*)
Sandwich box
Spirit level

Technique

1 Dissolve agarose at 10 mg/ml in Tris-barbital buffer pH 8.6 by heating
  in a microwave oven or on a stirring hotplate.

2 Pipette 5 ml of molten agarose on to a pre-coated glass slide on a
  level surface and allow to set. [1]

Notes

① See *Figure 5*, p. 44.

② Set up the electrophoresis apparatus according to manufacturer's instructions.

3 Cut two small holes in the agarose. ①

4 Fill an electrophoresis tank with Tris-barbital buffer pH 8.6. ②

5 Fill the wells in the gel with 10 μl of sample containing 1 μl of bromophenol blue. ③

6 Soak 3MM electrode strips in Tris-barbital buffer pH 8.6 and place one at each end of the slide.

7 Electrophorese the samples for ~1 h at 6 V/cm until the bromophenol blue nears the end of the slide.

8 Cut a trough in the agarose. ①

9 Fill the trough with 50 μl of specific antibody. ④

10 Leave overnight at RT in a humidified box. ②

11 Wash the gel extensively by very gentle agitation in six changes of distilled water over a period of 24 h.

12 Dry the gel overnight at RT by covering with two sheets of Whatman 3MM paper.

13 Peel off the 3MM paper and stain the gel by submerging in Coomassie brilliant blue staining solution for 5 min.

14 Destain by very gentle agitation in 5% methanol, 7% glacial acetic acid.

15 Examine the slide for bands of precipitation. ⑤

③ Sample might be serum, cell lysate, or any other mixture of antigens. Some gel punches produce smaller wells (e.g. 5 μl).

④ This might be against an antigen of interest or might be anti-immunoglobulin if analyzing serum immunoglobulins.

⑤ If required, the gel can be re-dried by placing between sheets of 3MM paper with a weight on top.

Pause points

1 Can be kept in a humidified box at 4°C for 2–3 days if necessary.

2 Can be kept in a humidified box at 4°C for 2–3 days if necessary.

Protocol 14. Immunoelectrophoresis

Protocol 15. Crossed (two-dimensional) electrophoresis

Reagents

Agarose (EEO ≥ 0.3)
Antibody solution
Antigen solution
0.05% (v/v) Coomassie brilliant blue R, in 50% methanol ⚠, 10% glacial acetic acid ⚠
Distilled water
7% Glacial acetic acid, in 5% methanol ⚠
Phosphate-buffered saline (PBS) pH 7.4
Tris-barbital buffer pH 8.6

Equipment

Absorbent paper towel
Beaker (e.g. 100 ml)
3MM chromatography paper (Whatman)
Electrophoresis tank (e.g. Multiphor II, Pharmacia)
Gel punch
Leveling tray
Microwave or stirring hotplate
Orbital shaker
Pipettes (e.g. 0.5–10 μl and 5 ml)
Pipette tips
Power pack
Pre-coated glass slides (*Protocol 11*)
Spirit level

Technique

1 Dissolve agarose at 10 mg/ml in Tris-barbital buffer pH 8.6 by heating in a microwave oven or on a stirring hotplate.

2 Pipette 5 ml of molten agarose on to a pre-coated glass slide on a level surface and allow to set. [1]

3 Cut two small holes, one at each end of the slide. ①

4 Fill an electrophoresis tank with Tris-barbital buffer pH 8.6. ②

Notes

① See *Figure 6*, p. 45.

② Set up the electrophoresis apparatus according to manufacturer's instructions.

③ Some gel punches produce smaller wells (e.g. 5 μl).

④ If required, the gel can be re-dried by placing between sheets of 3MM paper with a weight on top.

5 Fill the well nearest the anode with 10 µl of antibody and the well nearest the cathode with 10 µl of antigen. ③

6 Soak 3MM electrode strips in Tris-barbital buffer pH 8.6 and place one at each end of slide.

7 Electrophorese the samples for 30 min at 8 V/cm.

8 Wash the gel extensively by very gentle agitation in six changes of distilled water over a period of 24 h.

9 Dry the gel overnight at RT by covering with two sheets of 3MM paper.

10 Peel off the 3MM paper and stain the gel by submerging in Coomassie brilliant blue staining solution for 5 min.

11 Destain by very gentle agitation in 5% methanol, 7% glacial acetic acid.

12 Examine the slide for bands of precipitation. ④

Pause point

1 Can be kept in a humidified box at 4°C for 2–3 days if necessary.

Protocol 15. Crossed (two-dimensional) electrophoresis

Agglutination *(Protocols 16 and 17)*

Hemagglutination is a well established technique for detecting antigens present on the surface of erythrocytes (e.g. blood group determinants). However, it is also possible to couple nonerythrocyte antigens on to the red cells using a variety of reagents (for example chromic chloride, glutaraldehyde or tannic acid). Due to antibody bivalency, erythrocytes will be cross-linked in the presence of specific antibody leading to agglutination. When the procedure is carried out in U-bottom microtiter plates the agglutination can be seen as a 'mat' of cells, whereas in the absence of agglutination the erythrocytes will roll down to the bottom of the well and form a tight pellet of cells. The first protocol below provides a method for coupling antigen on to erythrocytes using chromic chloride. Erythrocytes coated with antigen using this technique can be used in both immunoagglutination (*Protocol 17*) and hemolytic plaque assays.

Protocol 16. **Conjugation of antigen to erythrocytes**

Reagents

Antigen
Chromic chloride (hexahydrate) ⚠
Buffer: phosphate-buffered saline (PBS) pH 7.4 containing 1% bovine serum albumin (BSA) and 0.1% sodium azide ⚠
Sheep red blood cells (SRBC) in Alsever's solution ⚠
0.15 M NaCl

Equipment

Centrifuge
Centrifuge tube, 50 ml polypropylene
Pipettes (e.g. 1 ml and 10 ml)
Pipette tips
Water bath

Technique

1 Pellet 10 ml of SRBC by centrifugation at 300 *g* for 5 min. ①

2 Discard the supernatant and resuspend pelleted SRBC in 50 ml of 0.15 M NaCl. Repeat centrifugation.

Notes

① SRBC provide a relatively inexpensive and convenient particle for antigen coating.

② Although a shaking water bath is most convenient, the tech-

3 Repeat step 2 three more times.

4 Add 1 ml of 2 mg/ml of antigen in 0.15 M NaCl to 1 ml of packed SRBC.

5 Slowly add 10 ml of freshly prepared 100 µg/ml chromic chloride in 0.15 M NaCl, whilst constantly shaking the tube.

6 Shake the tube gently in a water bath at 30°C for 40 min. ②

7 Pellet the SRBC by centrifugation at 300 g for 5 min.

8 Discard the supernatant and resuspend the pelleted SRBC in 50 ml of buffer. Repeat centrifugation.

9 Repeat step 8 twice more.

10 Resuspend the antigen-conjugated SRBC in 10 ml of buffer. ③

nique works perfectly well when using an ordinary water bath if the tube is inverted by hand every 5 min to distribute the SRBC evenly.

③ The antigen-conjugated SRBC will keep for up to 1 week at 4°C.

Protocol 16. Conjugation of antigen to erythrocytes

Protocol 17. **Immunoagglutination**

Reagents

Antibody
Antigen-conjugated erythrocytes (see *Protocol 16*)
Phosphate-buffered saline (PBS) containing 10% bovine serum albumin (BSA)

Equipment

Pipettes (e.g. 5–40 μl and 40–200 μl)
Pipette tips
96-well U-bottom microtiter plates

Technique

1 Place 75 μl of PBS containing 10% BSA into required number of wells of a U-bottom microtiter plate. ①

2 Add 25 μl of antibody to the first well of the row and mix thoroughly by taking the sample up and down several times in the pipette tip. Transfer 25 μl from well 1 to well 2. Continue sequential dilutions across the row to give fourfold dilutions of test antibody. ②

3 Add 25 μl/well of antigen-conjugated SRBC to each well and mix the contents of the wells thoroughly by tapping the sides of the plate. ③

4 Leave the plate at RT for 1 h on a level vibration-free surface.

5 Examine the wells for agglutination. ④

Notes

① Use one row to test each antibody sample.

② Alternatively other dilution series can be made, e.g. twofold by sequentially adding and removing 75 μl to 75 μl throughout the row.

③ Do not do this too vigorously or the contents will spill out of the wells.

④ A titer can be obtained, for comparative purposes, by identifying the highest dilution of antibody that is still able to produce agglutination.

IV DETECTION AND QUANTIFICATION OF CELL-ASSOCIATED ANTIGEN OR ANTIBODY

Cell surface and intracellular antigens can be detected using a variety of procedures, many of which are similar to those used for the detection of soluble antigens. Enzyme-labeled antibodies can be used for immunohistochemistry of tissue sections, and fluorochrome-labeled antibodies for immunofluorescence of both tissue sections and cell suspensions. In the case of cell suspensions, staining of viable cells will only result in the detection of cell surface-associated antigens because antibodies do not readily enter living cells. However, if the cells are first fixed and permeabilized, intracellular antigens can also be detected. Additionally, cells can be pelleted on to glass slides using a cytocentrifuge and then stained as for tissue sections. The secreted products of cells (e.g. antibodies, cytokines) can be measured using the enzyme-linked immunospot (ELISPOT) assay.

Methods available

Immunofluorescence (see *Protocols 18–22*)
General method for cell suspensions, adherent cell monolayers, cytocentrifuge preparations and tissue sections. Allows assignment of antigens to individual cells. Can be used for intracellular antigens following permeabilization of cells. Confocal microscopy permits greater resolution than that achieved by conventional fluorescence microscopy. Intracellular immunoglobulin in plasma cells can be detected using fluorochrome-labeled anti-immunoglobulin [1–5].
Problems: Requires fluorescence microscope or flow cytometer. Fluorescence fades with prolonged exposure of the sample under the fluo-

References

1. Coons, A.H. and Kaplan, M.H. (1950) *J. Exp. Med.* **91**, 1–13.
2. Johnson, G.D., Davidson, R.S., McNamee, K.C., Russell, G., Goodwin, D. and Holborow, E.J. (1982) *J. Immunol. Methods* **55**, 231–242.
3. Shapiro, H.M. (1988) *Practical Flow Cytometry*. Wiley-Liss, New York.
4. Loken, M.R. and Lanier, L.L. (1984) *Cytometry* **5**, 151–158.
5. Festin, R., Björklund, B. and Tötterman, T.H. (1987) *J. Immunol. Methods* **101**, 23–28.
6. Avrameas, S. (1972) *Histochem. J.* **4**, 321–330.

rescence microscope. With cell suspensions, capping and subsequent shedding or internalization of cell surface antigens may occur. This can be avoided by carrying out all procedures at 4°C in the presence of 0.1% sodium azide.

Immunohistochemistry (see *Protocols 23* and *24*)
A good method for the detection of cell-associated antigens in tissue sections, which can also be stained with histological dyes to aid characterization of the cells. The signal does not fade as with immunofluorescence and therefore the section can be examined for a longer period of time if necessary [6–9].
Problems: Although it allows assignment of antigens to individual cells in tissue sections, the degree of precision is not as good as immunofluorescence, especially if using fluorescence confocal microscopy. Endogenous enzyme activity within the tissue being examined can present problems.

Immunogold
Allows very precise localization of antigen within cells and tissues when combined with electron microscopy. Different sizes of gold particles can be attached to two or three different antibody specificities in order to co-localize antigens to particular cellular locations. Can also be used for light microscopy, particularly in conjunction with silver enhancing methods [10–14].
Problems: For ultrastructural studies access to an electron microscope is required.

7. Beesley, J.E. (ed.) (1993) *Immunocytochemistry: a Practical Approach*. IRL Press, Oxford.
8. Farr, A.G. and Nakane, P.K. (1981) *J. Immunol. Methods* **47**, 129–144.
9. Jones, E.L. and Gregory, J. (1989) in *Antibodies: a Practical Approach* (D. Catty, ed.), Vol II, pp. 155–177. IRL Press, Oxford, UK.
10. Guagliardi, L.E., Koppelman, B., Blum, J.S. *et al.* (1990) *Nature* **343**, 133–139.
11. Faulk, W. and Taylor, G. (1971) *Immunochemistry* **8**, 1081–1083.
12. Moeremans, M., Daneels, G., Van Dijck, A., Langanger, G. and De Mey, J. (1984) *J. Immunol. Methods* **74**, 353–360.
13. Bendayan, M. (1993) in *Practical Microscopy: a Beginner's Guide* (E. Hunter, ed.). 2nd Edn. pp. 71–92. Cambridge University Press, Cambridge, UK.
14. Polak, J.M. and Varndell, I.M. (eds) (1984) *Immunolabelling for Electron Microscopy*. Elsevier, Amsterdam.
15. Jerne, N.K. and Nordin, A.A. (1963) *Science* **140**, 405.
16. Cunningham, A.J. (1965) *Nature* **207**, 1106–1107.
17. Molinaro. G,A,, Eby, W.C. and Molinaro, C.A. (1981) *Methods Enzymol.* **73**, 326–338.
18. Sedgwick, J.D. and Holt, P.G. (1983) *J. Immunol. Methods* **57**, 301–309
19. Czerkinsky, C., Nilsson, L.Å., Nygren, H., Ouchterlony, Ö. and Tarkowski, A. (1983) *J. Immunol. Methods* **65**, 109–121.

Hemolytic plaque assays

The direct plaque assay uses antigen-coated erythrocytes to detect individual plasma cells secreting antibody of a defined antigen specificity. The indirect assay relies on anti-immunoglobulin-coated erythrocytes to detect all the cells secreting antibody of a given class or subclass, irrespective of antigen specificity [15–17].

Problems: Rather fiddly to set up.

ELISPOT (see Protocol 25)

An ELISA-based alternative to plaque assays. Antibody secreted from cultured lymphocytes is captured directly by antigen or anti-immunoglobulin coated onto a plastic surface such as a tissue culture plate. The ELISPOT assay can also be used to detect cytokine-secreting lymphocytes [18–20].

Problems: Uneven distribution of cells if the incubator is not absolutely level. nonspecific spots leading to overestimates of positive cells.

Choice of method

Immunofluorescence for both isolated cells and for tissue sections, with immunohistochemistry as an alternative assay for tissue sections. ELISPOT for detection of secreted cell products, particularly antibody.

20. Taguchi, T., McGee, J.R., Coffman, R.L., Beagley, K.W., Eldridge, J.H., Takasu, K. and Kiyono, H. (1990) *J. Immunol. Methods* **128**, 65–73.
21. Festin, R., Björklund, B. and Tötterman, T.H. (1987) *J. Immunol. Methods* **101**, 23–28.

Protocols provided

18. *Cell surface immunofluorescence*
19. *Cytocentrifuge preparations*
20. *Intracellular immunofluorescence on cytocentrifuge preparations*
21. *Intracellular immunofluorescence on cell suspensions*
22. *Immunofluorescence on tissue sections*
23. *Dewaxing and clearing of paraffin-embedded tissue sections*
24. *Enzyme-linked immunohistochemistry*
25. *Enzyme-linked immunospot (ELISPOT)*

Immunofluorescence (*Protocols 18–22*)

A major advantage of immunofluorescence is that two or more parameters can be measured simultaneously, most commonly using FITC-labeled antibody against one antigen and TRITC, PE or TR-labeled antibody against a second antigen. Two-color fluorescence is equally applicable to cell suspensions and tissue sections. Triple antibody binding can be detected on cell suspensions using three-color fluorescence with dual laser flow cytometry [4] or two-color fluorescence and immunogold with a single laser [21].

For the staining procedure itself, although tubes are more tedious to handle than microtiter plates, the latter are more prone to cross-contamination between wells. The likelihood of this occurring can be reduced by leaving empty wells surrounding those that are used. After the washing steps, the removal of the buffer is most easily achieved using a disposable pipette tip attached to a vacuum line. Cell losses are minimized by gentle handling of the tubes or plates.

Nonantigen-specific binding to Fc receptors can lead to false positive results, but this can be minimized by centrifugation of the antibody at 100 000 g for 15 min prior to use, by competitively blocking the binding with serum (or for mouse leukocytes, with Fc Block™, PharMingen), or by the use of Fab or $F(ab)_2$ fragments of the antibodies. Isotype-matched negative controls should be included in every assay. Dead cells may also stain nonspecifically with antibodies. The addition of 1 μl of ethidium bromide △ or propidium iodide △ (50 μg/ml in PBS) to the resuspended cells prior to examination under the fluorescence microscope is therefore useful in distinguishing dead cells, the nuclei of which are stained by these dyes. Cells can be fixed by resuspension in 1% paraformaldehyde △ following staining and may then be stored for up to 1 week before analysis. Note, however, that cells stained with ethidium bromide or propidium iodide should not be fixed as the dyes then diffuse into the viable cells.

When incubating reagents on glass slide preparations of cells or tissues it is extremely important that the slides are not allowed to dry out at any stage, as this will lead to nonspecific binding. A perfectly adequate humidified box can be made by placing a well-dampened tissue in a container such as a sandwich box. Make sure the lid is firmly replaced after placing slides in the box. Do not blot slides dry or leave them for longer than 15 sec without the tissue sections or cell spots being covered with reagent. To prevent the antibody solution spreading, ensure the glass immediately surrounding the tissue sections or cell spots is perfectly dry. Multi-spot slides which have several spots separated by a Teflon coating are particularly useful if several tissue sections are to be examined.

Immunofluorescence on cytocentrifuge preparations can be used to detect intracellular antigens and is a commonly used method for analyzing the isotype of immunoglobulins within plasma cells. In the latter case it can be carried out as a direct assay, following *Protocol 20* but omitting steps 4–8. When analysing lymphocytes it is essential that the combination of antibodies chosen is such that the fluoro-chrome-labeled anti-immunoglobulin will not detect the membrane immunoglobulin on the B-cells, unless this is the aim of the experiment.

Cell-associated antigen or antibody

Protocol 18. **Cell surface immunofluorescence**

Reagents

Anti-quench reagent (e.g. 1,4-diazobicyclo-[2.2.2]-octane, DABCO) ⚠

Fluorochrome-labeled anti-immunoglobulin (reactive with the primary antibody but not against the immunoglobulin of the species whose cells are being used)

Nail polish

Paraformaldehyde ⚠ , 1% (10 mg/ml in 0.15 M NaCl pH 7.4, warmed to aid solubility)

Buffer: phosphate-buffered saline (PBS) pH 7.4 containing 1% bovine serum albumin (BSA) and 0.1% sodium azide ⚠

Primary antibody (specific for cell surface antigen)

Equipment

Centrifuge

Cover slips (22 × 22 mm, thickness No. 1)

Fluorescent microscope or flow cytometer

Glass slides (76 × 26 mm)

Ice bucket

Pipettes (e.g. 5–40 μl, 40–200 μl and 1–5 ml)

Pipette tips

12 × 15 mm round bottom test tubes or 96-well U-bottom microtiter plates

Vortex mixer

Technique

1 Centrifuge 2×10^5 cells at 300 *g* for 7 min in tubes or U-bottom microtiter plates.

2 Remove virtually all the buffer.

3 Gently resuspend the cells in the residual buffer using a vortex mixer and then add 30 µl of cold (4°C) buffer.

4 Add 30 µl of a predetermined optimal concentration of primary antibody in cold buffer. ①

Notes

① Note that at this step the antibody becomes diluted 1 in 2.

② Fully frozen ice does not make good contact with the plastic but make sure it is not melting to the extent that the tubes sink below the surface.

③ If using a flow cytometer for analysis, the cells should be resuspended in 200 μl of cold incubation buffer and kept on melting ice until analyzed. For flow cytometry the anti-quench agent is unnecessary as in this case the fluoro-

5 Put the tubes/plate on melting ice for 30 min. ②

6 Add 2 ml (for test tubes) or 100 µl (for microtiter plate wells) of cold buffer and centrifuge at 300 *g* for 7 min at 4°C.

7 Remove the buffer and resuspend the cells in residual buffer. Repeat the wash step once for test tubes and three times for microtiter plates by adding more cold buffer followed by centrifugation.

8 Resuspend the cells in 30 µl of cold buffer as in step 3.

9 Add 30 µl of a predetermined optimal concentration of fluorochrome-labeled anti-immunoglobulin in cold incubation buffer and keep on melting ice for 30 min. ①

10 Wash the cells as above (steps 6–7).

11 Resuspend the cells in the residual buffer and add 20 µl of cold buffer containing anti-quench reagent. ③

12 To examine the cells under a fluorescence microscope, place the cells on a glass slide, cover with a cover slip, and seal with nail polish.

chromes are only excited for a very short period of time. If the cells are not to be analyzed straight away (<1 h) they should be resuspended in 1% paraformaldehyde and placed at 4°C until analyzed (within 1–2 days).

Protocol 19. Cytocentrifuge preparations

Reagents

5% Glacial acetic acid, in ethanol ⚠
Buffer: phosphate-buffered saline (PBS) containing 5% bovine serum albumin (BSA)

Equipment

Absorbent paper towel
Coplin jars
Cytocentrifuge (e.g. Shandon cytospin 2)
Cytocentrifuge filter cards
Diamond point marker
Glass slides (76 × 26 mm)
Pipettes (e.g. 40–200 μl and 1–5 ml)
Pipette tips

Technique

1 Adjust the cell concentration to 2.5×10^5/ml in buffer.

2 Label clean microscope slides using a diamond point marker.

3 Place the slides and cytocentrifuge filter cards in the cytocentrifuge.

4 Place 100 μl of cell suspension in each sample chamber.

5 Centrifuge at 32 g for 10 min.

6 Carefully remove the slides and filter cards and place the slides cell-side up on to a paper towel. ①

7 Allow the slides to air dry. ② 1

Notes

① The filter cards can be dried and re-used four or five times.

② Either on the laboratory bench or on racks in a drying oven.

8 Fix the cells by immersing the slides in 5% glacial acetic acid in ethanol for 20 min at −20°C.

9 Air dry the slides.

Pause point

1 Slides can be stored for several months in an air-tight container at −70°C.

Protocol 19. Cytocentrifuge preparations

Reagents

Buffer: phosphate-buffered saline (PBS) containing 1% bovine serum albumin (BSA)

Fixed cytocentrifuge preparations

Fluorochrome-labeled anti-immunoglobulin (reactive with the primary antibody but not against the immunoglobulin of the species whose cells are being used)

Mounting medium: e.g. 1,4 diazabicyclo-[2.2.2]-octane (DABCO) glycerol ⚠

Phosphate-buffered saline (PBS) pH 7.4

Primary antibody (specific for antigen of interest)

Equipment

Absorbent paper tissues

Coplin jars

Cover slips (22 × 22 mm, thickness No. 1)

Fluorescence microscope

Humidified chamber (e.g. sandwich box and wet tissue paper)

Magnetic stirrer and spin bar

Nail polish

Pipettes (e.g. 5–40 μl, 40–200 μl and 1–5 ml)

Pipette tips

Squirt bottle

Technique

1 Wash fixed slides by immersion in PBS, stirring gently with a magnetic spin bar. Wash for 30 min, changing the wash solution every 10 min.

2 Remove the slides one at a time from the PBS. Let excess PBS drain off and very carefully and quickly wipe the glass surrounding the cell spot. ①

3 Place the slides face up in a humidified chamber.

4 Cover the cell spots with 25 µl of a predetermined optimal concentration (see pp. 5, 6) of the primary antibody in buffer.

Notes

① Such that the glass slide becomes dry but the cell spot remains damp.

② Do not leave for longer than 15 sec from the time of removal from the PBS until addition of fluorochrome-labeled anti-immunoglobulin.

③ Do not leave for longer than 15 sec from the time of removal from the PBS until addition of mounting medium.

④ Lowered at an angle in order to avoid trapping air bubbles.

5 Incubate the slides in the humidified chamber for 30 min at RT.

6 Gently wash off the primary antibody using PBS from a squirt bottle.

7 Wash the slides by immersion in PBS, stirring gently with a magnetic spin bar. Wash for 30 min, changing the wash solution every 10 min.

8 Remove the slides one at a time from the PBS. Let excess PBS drain off and very carefully and quickly wipe the glass surrounding the cell spot. ②

9 Cover the cell spots with 25 μl of a predetermined optimal concentration (see pp. 5, 6) of fluorochrome-labeled anti-immunoglobulin in buffer.

10 Incubate the slides in the humidified chamber for 30 min at RT.

11 Gently wash off the labeled antibody using PBS from a squirt bottle.

12 Wash the slides with PBS, stirring gently with a magnetic spin bar. Wash for 30 min changing the wash solution every 10 min.

13 Remove the slides one at a time from the PBS. Let excess PBS drain off and very carefully and quickly wipe the glass surrounding the cell spot. ③

14 Place one drop of mounting medium on top of the cell spot and gently cover with a cover slip. ④ ☐1

15 Examine the slides using a fluorescence microscope.

Pause point

☐1 Slides can be stored for several weeks at 4°C wrapped in foil.

                  Protocol 20. Intracellular immunofluorescence on cytocentrifuge preparations

Protocol 21. Intracellular immunofluorescence on cell suspensions

Reagents

Anti-quench reagent (e.g. 1,4-diazobicyclo-[2.2.2]-octane, DABCO) ⚠

Cell suspension (⚠)

Fluorochrome-labeled anti-immunoglobulin (reactive with the primary antibody but not against the immunoglobulin of the species whose cells are being used)

Nail polish

2% Paraformaldehyde ⚠ in 0.1 M phosphate buffer pH 7.4

Buffer: phosphate-buffered saline (PBS) pH 7.4 containing 1% bovine serum albumin (BSA), 0.1% sodium azide ⚠

Phosphate-buffered saline (PBS) pH 7.4

Primary antibody (specific for antigen of interest)

0.06% Saponin ⚠ in 0.1% ovalbumin, 0.1 mM glycine in PBS

Equipment

Centrifuge

Cover slips (22 × 22 mm, thickness No. 1)

Glass slides (76 × 26 mm)

Fluorescence microscope or flow cytometer

Pipettes (e.g. 5–40 μl, 40–200 μl, 1–5 ml)

Pipette tips

12 × 15 mm round bottom test tubes or 96-well U-bottom microtiter plates

Vortex mixer

Technique

1 Centrifuge 2 × 10^5 cells at 4°C at 300 g for 7 min in tubes or U-bottom microtiter plates.

2 Remove virtually all the buffer.

3 Gently resuspend cells in residual buffer using a vortex mixer and then add 200 µl 2% paraformaldehyde in 0.1 M phosphate buffer pH 7.4.

4 Incubate for 20 min at 4°C.

5 Centrifuge the cells at 300 g for 7 min at RT.

6 Discard the supernatant and resuspend the cells in 200 µl of PBS.[1]

Notes

① If using a flow cytometer for analysis, the cells should be resuspended in 200 μl of incubation buffer. For flow cytometry the anti-quench agent is unnecessary as in this case the fluorochromes are only excited for a very short period of time.

7 Centrifuge the cells at 300 g for 7 min at RT.

8 Discard the supernatant and resuspend the cells in 200 µl of 0.06% saponin, 0.1% ovalbumin, 0.1 mM glycine in PBS.

9 Leave for 20 min at RT.

10 Centrifuge the cells at 300 g for 7 min, discard the supernatant and then resuspend the cells in 30 µl of a predetermined optimal concentration of primary antibody in buffer.

11 Leave for 30 min at RT.

12 Add 2 ml (for test tubes) or 100 µl (for microtiter plate wells) of buffer and centrifuge at 300 g for 7 min at RT.

13 Remove the buffer and resuspend the cells in residual buffer. Repeat the wash step once for test tubes and three times for microtiter plates by adding more buffer followed by centrifugation.

14 Resuspend the cells in 30 µl of a predetermined optimal concentration of fluorochrome-labeled anti-immunoglobulin in buffer and leave for 30 min at RT.

15 Wash the cells as above (Steps 12–13).

16 Resuspend the cells in residual buffer and add 20 µl of buffer containing anti-quench reagent. ①

17 To examine the slides using a fluorescence microscope, place the cells on a glass slide, cover with a cover slip and seal with nail polish.

Pause point

1 Cells can be stored at 4°C for several days if the PBS contains 0.1% sodium azide. ⚠

Protocol 21. Intracellular immunofluorescence on cell suspensions

Protocol 22. Immunofluorescence on tissue sections

Reagents

Buffer: 1% bovine serum albumin (BSA), 0.1% sodium azide ⚠ in PBS pH 7.4

Fluorochrome-labeled anti-immunoglobulin (reactive with the primary antibody but not against the immunoglobulin of the species whose tissue is being used)

Methanol ⚠

Mounting medium: 1,4 diazabicyclo-[2.2.2]-octane (DABCO) glycerol ⚠

Nail polish

Phosphate-buffered saline (PBS) pH 7.4

Primary antibody (specific for antigen of interest)

Tissue sections on glass microscope slides

Equipment

Absorbent paper tissues

Cover slips (22 × 50 mm, thickness number 1)

Cryostat

Fluorescence microscope

Humidified chamber (e.g. sandwich box and wet tissue paper)

Magnetic stirrer and spin bar

Pipettes (e.g. 5–40 μl, 40–200 μl and 1–5 ml)

Pipette tips

Squirt bottle

Washing dish and rack

Technique

1 Cut 4–6 μm tissue sections on a cryostat and transfer each section immediately on to a scrupulously clean glass slide.

2 Air dry the slides. ① 1

3 Fix the slides by immersion in methanol for 3 min. ② 2

4 Wash the slides with PBS, stirring gently with a magnetic spin bar. Wash for 30 min changing the wash solution every 10 min.

Notes

① Either on the laboratory bench or on racks in a drying oven.

② For some tissue antigens alternative fixatives may be required, e.g. acetone. ⚠

③ So that the glass slide becomes dry but the tissue section remains damp.

④ Lower cover slip at an angle in order to avoid trapping air bubbles.

5　Remove the slides one at a time from the PBS. Very carefully and quickly wipe the glass surrounding each section. ③

6　Place the slides face up in a humidified chamber.

7　Cover the tissue sections with 25 µl of a predetermined optimal concentration of the primary antibody in buffer.

8　Incubate the slides in the humidified chamber for 30 min at RT.

9　Very gently wash off the primary antibody using PBS from a squirt bottle.

10　Wash the slides with PBS, stirring gently with a magnetic spin bar. Wash for 30 min, changing the wash solution every 10 min.

11　Remove the slides one at a time from the PBS. Very carefully and quickly wipe the glass surrounding each section. ③

12　Cover the tissue sections with 25 µl of a predetermined optimal concentration of fluorochrome-labeled anti-immunoglobulin in buffer.

13　Incubate the slides in the humidified chamber for 30 min at RT.

14　Very gently wash off the antibody using PBS from a squirt bottle.

15　Wash the slides with PBS, stirring gently with a magnetic spin bar. Wash for 30 min changing the wash solution every 10 min.

16　Remove the slides one at a time from the PBS. Very carefully and quickly wipe the glass surrounding each section. ③

Continued overleaf

Protocol 22. Immunofluorescence on tissue sections

17 Place one drop of mounting medium on top of each tissue section and gently cover with a cover slip. Seal with nail polish. ④ ③

18 Examine the slides using a fluorescence microscope.

Pause points

1. Slides can be stored for several months in an air-tight container at −70°C.

2. Slides can be stored for several months in an air-tight container at −70°C.

3. Slides can be stored for several weeks at 4°C wrapped in foil.

Enzyme-linked assays for cell-associated antigens *(Protocols 23–25)*

The use of enzyme-linked antibodies to detect antigens in tissue sections has the advantage over fluorochrome-labeled antibodies in that the section can be examined at length using conventional bright field microscopy, and the tissue sections can be counter-stained with histological dyes to aid identification of the cells. In addition to fixation, some antigens may need to be 'unmasked' (e.g. using mild proteolytic enzyme treatment) before they can be detected by immunohistochemistry. Amplification techniques are available such as the peroxidase–anti-peroxidase (PAP) and alkaline phosphatase–anti-alkaline phosphatase (APAAP) procedures for cases where a higher degree of sensitivity is required.

Although, as with immunofluorescence, these techniques are perhaps most easily carried out on cryostat-produced tissue sections, it is often the case that histological tissue sections are embedded in paraffin. In this instance they must first be dewaxed prior to staining, as described in *Protocol 23*. The enzyme-linked immunohistochemistry protocol provided (*Protocol 24*) can be applied to cell smears and imprints as well as to tissue sections. Endogenous enzyme activity within the tissue being examined can sometimes present problems. If this should prove to be the case it is usually best to change to a different enzyme label (e.g. β-galactosidase) on the antibody, but another option is to block the endogenous enzyme activity. Peroxidase activity can be blocked by incubating the specimen with 0.1% phenylhydrazine hydrochloride in PBS for 20 min, and alkaline phosphatase activity by the addition of 0.1 mM levamisole to the substrate solution.

The enzyme-linked immunospot assay (*Protocol 25*) permits the detection of the products of viable cells in culture, such as antibody secreted by B cells or cytokines secreted by T cells or other cell types. In the latter instance, cytokine-specific antibody is immobilized on the plastic surface. As with enzyme-linked immunohistochemistry, the basis of the assay is the generation of an insoluble colored product of an enzyme reaction.

Cell-associated antigen or antibody

Protocol 23. Dewaxing and clearing of paraffin-embedded tissue

Reagents

Ethanol ⚠
Phosphate-buffered saline (PBS) pH 7.4
Tissue section slides from paraffin-embedded tissue
Xylene ⚠

Equipment

Coplin jars
Oven (56°C)

Technique

1 Place the tissue section slides in a 56°C oven for 20 min. ①

2 Transfer the slides to a Coplin jar containing xylene and leave at RT for 5 min.

3 Pour off the xylene and replace with fresh xylene for a further 5 min.

4 Transfer the slides to a Coplin jar containing absolute ethanol and leave for 3 min.

5 Pour off the ethanol and replace with fresh absolute ethanol for a further 3 min.

6 Transfer the slides to a Coplin jar containing 90% ethanol and leave for 3 min.

7 Transfer the slides to a Coplin jar containing 80% ethanol and leave for 3 min.

Notes

① Temperature must not exceed 60°C.

② Air-dried slides can be stored for several months in an air-tight container at –70°C.

8 Transfer the slides to a Coplin jar under gently running tap water for 30 sec.

9 Either air dry the slides or proceed to step 4 of *Protocol 24*. ②

Protocol 24. Enzyme-linked immunohistochemistry

Reagents

Buffer: 1% bovine serum albumin (BSA) in PBS pH 7.4
Horseradish peroxidase (HRP)-labeled anti-immunoglobulin (reactive with the primary antibody but not against the immunoglobulin of the species whose tissue is being used)
30% Hydrogen peroxide ⚠
Methanol ⚠
Mounting medium (e.g. Gelvatol, Monsanto Chemicals)
Nail polish
Phosphate-buffered saline (PBS) pH 7.4
Primary antibody (specific for antigen of interest)
Substrate: 6 mg of diaminobenzidine tetrahydrochloride ⚠(DAB) in 10 ml of 0.05 M Tris-HCl buffer pH 7.6
Tissue sections on glass microscope slides

Equipment

Absorbent paper tissues
Cover slips (22 × 50 mm, thickness number 1)
Cryostat
Humidified chamber (e.g. sandwich box and wet tissue paper)
Magnetic stirrer and spin bar
Microscope
Pipettes (e.g. 5–40 μl, 40–200 μl, 200–1000 μl and 1–5 ml)
Pipette tips
Squirt bottle
Washing dish and rack

Technique

1 Cut 4–6 μm tissue sections on a cryostat and transfer each section immediately on to a clean glass slide. ①

2 Air dry the slides. 1

3 Rinse the slides in PBS and fix by immersion in methanol for 3 min. ② 2

Notes

① Alternatively use dewaxed and cleared paraffin sections (see *Protocol 23*) and begin the staining procedure at step 4.

② For some tissue antigens alternative fixatives may be required, for example acetone. ⚠

③ If it is necessary to eliminate endogenous tissue peroxidase activity, cover the section with 100 μl of 0.1% phenyl-

4 Rinse the slides in PBS and place face up in a humidified chamber. ③

5 Cover the tissue sections with 100 µl of a predetermined optimal concentration (see pp. 5, 6) of the primary antibody in buffer.

6 Incubate the slides in the humidified chamber for 30 min at RT.

7 Gently wash off the primary antibody using PBS from a squirt bottle.

8 Wash the slides with PBS, stirring gently with a magnetic spin bar. Wash for 15 min, changing the wash solution every 5 min.

9 Remove the slides one at a time from the PBS. Very carefully and quickly wipe the glass surrounding each section. ④

10 Cover the tissue sections with 100 µl of a predetermined optimal concentration of HRP-labeled anti-immunoglobulin in buffer. ⑤

11 Incubate the slides in the humidified chamber for 30 min at RT.

12 Gently wash off the labeled antibody using PBS from a squirt bottle.

13 Wash the slides with PBS, stirring gently with a magnetic spin bar. Wash for 15 min, changing the wash solution every 5 min.

14 Remove the slides one at a time from the PBS. Very carefully and quickly wipe the glass surrounding each section. ④

15 Cover the tissue sections with 100 µl of DAB substrate. ⑥

hydrazine hydrochloride ⚠ in PBS for 20 min at RT and then wash off with PBS from a squirt bottle followed by two 2-min washes in PBS.

④ So that the glass slide becomes dry but the tissue section remains damp.

⑤ Alternatively alkaline phosphatase- or β-galactosidase-labeled anti-immunoglobulin can be used.

⑥ Add 10 μl of 30% H_2O_2 to 10 ml of DAB substrate immediately prior to use. For alkaline phosphatase-labeled antibodies use 5-bromo-4-chloro-3-indolyl phosphate (BCIP) nitro blue tetrazolium (NBT) ⚠ substrate (e.g. Sigma FAST BCIP/NBT tablets), for β-galactosidase-labeled antibodies use 5-bromo-4-chloro-3-indolyl-β-D-galactopyranoside (BCIG) ⚠ substrate.

⑦ The incubation time can be adjusted to vary the intensity of substrate formed (usually between 5 and 30 min is optimal).

⑧ At this stage the slide can be counterstained with a histological stain if so desired (e.g. hematoxylin ⚠ for 5 min at RT followed by a 5-min wash under gently running tap water). The alkaline phosphatase reaction is more efficiently stopped if 20 mM EDTA is added to the PBS.

⑨ Lower cover slip at an angle in order to avoid trapping air bubbles.

Continued overleaf

Protocol 24. Enzyme-linked immunohistochemistry

16 Incubate in the humidified chamber at RT for 20 min. ⑦

17 Gently wash the slides using PBS from a squirt bottle. ⑧

18 Very carefully and quickly wipe the glass surrounding each section. ④

19 Place one drop of aqueous mounting medium on top of the tissue section and gently cover with a cover slip. Seal with nail polish. ⑨

20 Examine the slides under a microscope.

Pause points

1 Slides can be stored for several months in an air-tight container at –70°C.

2 Slides can be stored for several months in an air-tight container at –70°C.

Cell-associated antigen or antibody

Protocol 25. **Enzyme-linked immunospot (ELISPOT)**

Reagents

Agarose
Antibody-secreting cells (e.g. spleen cells from an immunized mouse)
Antigen
Bovine serum albumin (BSA), 1% in PBS (blocking agent)
Dimethylsulfoxide (DMSO) ⚠
4% Dried skimmed milk powder (e.g. Marvel) in 0.05% Tween 20 in PBS (ELISA buffer)
Horseradish peroxidase (HRP)-labeled anti-immunoglobulin
30% Hydrogen peroxide ⚠
Phosphate-buffered saline (PBS) pH 7.4
Sodium acetate, 0.1 M pH 6.0
12% Sulfuric acid ⚠

Tetramethylbenzidine (TMB) ⚠
Tissue culture medium (e.g. RPMI 1640 containing 10% heat-inactivated fetal calf serum (HIFCS) and antibiotics)
0.05% Tween 20 in PBS (PBS-T)

Equipment

37°C CO_2 incubator
Microscope
Pipettes (e.g., 5–40 μl, 40–200 μl, 200–1000 μl and 1–5 ml)
Pipette tips
Squirt bottle
24-well polystyrene tissue culture plate

Technique

1 Place 500 µl of antigen at 10 µg/ml in PBS into each well of a polystyrene tissue culture plate. Replace the lid and leave overnight at 4°C. ①

2 Wash the wells of the plate three times with PBS.

3 Add 1 ml/well of 1% BSA in PBS and incubate for 1 h at RT. ☐1

4 Wash the wells of the plate three times with PBS.

Notes

① Higher concentrations may give better results with some antigens. For the detection of total immunoglobulin-secreting cells the wells should be coated with anti-immunoglobulin. For cytokine detection use a monoclonal antibody specific for the cytokine of interest.

② Individual experiments will differ in the optimal cell concentration (usually 10^4–10^6/ml) and optimal time of incubation

5 Add 500 μl/well of cells at 10^5/ml in tissue culture medium and incubate at 37°C in a CO_2 incubator for 16 h. ②

6 Remove the cells and wash the wells of the plate three times with PBS-T.

7 Add 500 μl/well of a predetermined optimal concentration of HRP-labeled anti-IgG in ELISA buffer and leave for 2 h at RT. ③

8 Wash the wells of the plate three times with PBS.

9 Add 200 μl/well of TMB substrate dissolved in agarose and then quickly flick off any excess before the gel sets. ④

10 Leave in the dark at RT for 2–16 h. ⑤

11 Count the number of strong, well-defined spots, using 10× magnification. ⑥

(usually 2–24 h). Controls should include wells coated with an irrelevant antigen or antibody. To confirm that *de novo* secretion is occurring, include 100 μg/ml cycloheximide ⚠ (an inhibitor of protein synthesis) in some of the wells during the cell culture. It is vital that the incubator is absolutely level to prevent cells rolling to one edge of the well.

③ The developing antibody used will depend on the parameter being measured, in this case IgG antibodies specific for the antigen coated on to the well. In other instances the antibody might be specific for a cytokine of interest.

④ Dissolve 0.1 mg of TMB in 100 μl of DMSO. Add to 9.9 ml of 12 mg/ml agarose in 0.1 M sodium acetate pH 6.0 (dissolved using a microwave and then cooled in a 46°C water bath) and then add 3.3 μl of 30% hydrogen peroxide immediately before use.

⑤ Until strong spots of enzyme substrate have developed.

⑥ Any small or faint spots are likely to be artefacts and should not be counted.

Pause point

1 The plate can be left at 4°C for several days if the blocking agent contains 0.1% sodium azide. ⚠

Protocol 25. Enzyme-linked immunospot (ELISPOT)

V PURIFICATION OF ANTIGEN OR ANTIBODY

Numerous techniques are used as purification procedures for proteins. Amongst the most powerful of these are immunoprecipitation and affinity chromatography, both of which exploit the exquisite specificity of the antibody molecule. These techniques routinely allow a greater than 1000-fold enrichment of the protein of interest. Critical parameters include the specificity of the antibody reagent and its affinity. The affinity should optimally be between 10^6 M^{-1} and 10^8 M^{-1} in free solution. Significantly lower affinity interactions may be insufficient for successful affinity chromatography or immunoprecipitation, whilst interactions of significantly higher affinity may present difficulties in eluting the protein from an affinity column without denaturation occurring.

Methods available

Gel filtration chromatography

Separates proteins on the basis of molecular size using porous gels of cross-linked dextran or agarose to create a molecular sieve of defined pore size [1–3].

Problems: Protein may be contaminated with other molecules of a similar size.

Ion-exchange chromatography

Separates proteins on the basis of their surface charge. Electrostatic binding on to a matrix bearing the opposite charge is followed by differential elution by either increasing the ionic strength or changing the pH of the buffer. Both cationic (e.g. carboxymethyl cellulose, CMC) and anionic (diethylaminoethyl cellulose, DEAE) matrices are available [4–7].

References

1. *Gel Filtration: Principles and Methods.* 6th edn. Pharmacia Biotech, Uppsala.
2. Fischer, L. (1980) *Gel Filtration Chromatography.* Elsevier. Amsterdam.
3. Sofer, G.K. and Nyström, L.E. (1991) *Process Chromatography: a Guide to Validation.* Academic Press. London.
4. *Ion Exchange Chromatography: Principles and Methods.* 3rd edn. Pharmacia Biotech, Uppsala.
5. Himmelhoch, S.R. (1971) *Methods Enzymol.* **22**, 273–286.
6. Jiskoot, W., Hoven, A.M. De Koning, A.A. Leerling, M.F. Reubsaet, C.H. Crommelin, D.J. and Beuvery, E.C. (1991) *J. Immunol Methods.* **138**, 181–189.
7. Krotkiewski, H. Gronberg, G. Krotkiewska, B. Nilsson, B. and Svensson, S. (1990) *J. Biol. Chem.* **265**, 20195–20201.

Problems: Protein may be contaminated with other molecules of similar surface charge.

Preparative isoelectric focusing
Separates proteins on the basis of their isoelectric points [8–10].
Problems: Protein may be contaminated with other molecules of a similar pI.

Affinity chromatography (see *Protocols 26–28*)
Separation based upon ligand-specific interaction, giving the potential for a very high level of specific enrichment [11–15].
Problems: Elution often requires fairly harsh conditions with the attendant potential for damage to the protein. Not suitable for use with very low or very high affinity antibodies, respectively, due to a lack of stable binding or inability to elute readily.

Immunoprecipitation (see *Protocols 29, 30*)
Ligand-specific interaction followed by precipitation of the complex using a second (precipitating) antibody or other agent such as fixed *Staphylococcus aureus* Cowan 1 (SAC) [16–18].
Problems: Dependent on antibody affinity. Affinities of lower than 10^6 M^{-1} will not usually produce satisfactory results. Nonspecific precipitation of irrelevant antigens is a common problem. Recovery of the antigen in the native state is not as straightforward as with affinity chromatography.

8. Evans, L.L. and Burns, M.A. (1995). *Bio/Technology* **13**, 46–52.
9. Nag, B., Arimilli, S., Koukis, B., Rhodes, E., Baichwal, V. and Sharma, S.D. (1994) *J. Biol. Chem.* **269**, 10061–10070.
10. Peritt, D., Flechner, I., Okunev, E., Yanai, P., Halperin, T., Treves, A.J. and Barak, V. (1992) *J. Immunol. Methods.* **155**, 159–165.
11. Dean, P.D.G., Johnson, W.S. and Middle, F.A. (eds) (1985) *Affinity Chromatography: a Practical Approach.* IRL Press, Oxford.
12. Wilchek, M., Miron, T. and Kohn, J. (1984) *Methods Enzymol.* **104**, 3–55.
13. Cuatrecasas, P. (1970) *Nature* **228**, 1327–1328.
14. *Affinity Chromatography: Principles and Methods.* Pharmacia Biotech, Uppsala.
15. Tsang, V.C.W. and Wilkins, P.P. (1991) *J. Immunol. Methods* **138**, 291–299.
16. Kessler, S.W. (1981) *Methods Enzymol.* **73**, 442–458.
17. Schlager, S.I. (1980) *Methods Enzymol.* **70**, 252–265.
18. Scheidtmann, K.H. (1989) in *Protein Structure: a Practical Approach.* (T.E. Creighton, ed.) IRL Press, Oxford, pp. 93–115.

Choice of method

Gel filtration is simple and quick, but affinity chromatography achieves the highest degree of specific enrichment combined with ease of recovery of the antigen in its native state.

Protocols provided

26. *Ligand immobilization on Sepharose beads*
27. *Immunoaffinity chromatography on columns*
28. *Batch immunoaffinity chromatography*
29. *Immunoprecipitation of fluid phase antigen*
30. *Immunoprecipitation of cellular antigens*

Affinity chromatography (*Protocols 26–28*)

Affinity chromatography permits rapid separations with a degree of antigen specificity unobtainable with any other method. The molecule to be purified is specifically, but reversibly, absorbed to an immobilized ligand on a solid support, permitting the concentration of dilute proteins from large volumes. The technique is extremely widely employed both in small-scale laboratory experimentation and for large-scale commercial purification processes. Protein A and protein G absorbents are available in pre-packed columns which are ideal for the purification of monoclonal antibodies. In cases where an antibody of a given specificity needs to be purified from a polyclonal antibody preparation, this can be achieved by coupling the antigen of interest to the beads.

One gram of dry Sepharose produces approximately 3.5 ml of gel. Washing of Sepharose beads prior to coupling is most easily achieved using a G3 pore size sintered glass filter attached to a vacuum flask. The gel is swirled for 3 min and then the vacuum applied. The wash solution drains out and can be replaced with fresh wash solution. The final wash solution is removed by vacuum until cracks begin to appear in the gel cake. The binding capacity of antigen-coated beads will differ for different antigens and may vary with each coupling reaction using the same antigen. If desired, the binding capacity can be determined empirically by addition of different amounts of the antibody to a set volume of antigen-coated beads. Although affinity chromatography is usually carried out in columns (*Protocol 27*), it can also be carried out, although usually less efficiently, as a batch procedure in test tubes (*Protocol 28*).

Protocol 26. Ligand immobilization on Sepharose beads

Reagents

0.1 M Acetate buffer, 0.5 M NaCl pH 4.0
Antigen
1 M Ethanolamine ⚠
1 mM HCl ⚠
0.1 M NaHCO$_3$, 0.5 M NaCl pH 8.3
Sepharose 4B, cyanogen bromide activated (Pharmacia)

Equipment

Centrifuge tube, 50 ml polypropylene
End-over-end rotary mixer (e.g. 10 r.p.m.)
Side-arm vacuum flask
Sintered glass funnel (50 ml capacity)

Technique

1 Resuspend the required amount of activated dry Sepharose in ice-cold 1 mM HCl (5 ml/g Sepharose) and transfer to a scintered glass filter.

2 Wash the Sepharose five times on the filter, each time for 3 min with 40 ml of ice-cold 1 mM HCl/g dry Sepharose.

3 Following removal of the final wash solution, transfer the Sepharose to a suitable tube and immediately add, for each ml of Sepharose, 2 ml of the protein to be coupled at 2.5 mg/ml in 0.1 M NaHCO$_3$, 0.5 M NaCl pH 8.3. ①

4 Leave for 2 h at RT in an end-over-end mixer at a fairly slow speed (e.g. 10 r.p.m). ② [1]

Notes

① IgG may couple more efficiently at a slightly higher pH, e.g. in 0.2 M NaHCO$_3$ 0.5 M NaCl pH 9.0.

② A gentle roller can also be used but magnetic stirrers should be avoided as they tend to damage the Sepharose beads.

③ Or 0.2 M glycine pH 8.0. These procedures block excess active groups.

④ The ligand-coupled gel can be stored for many months at 4°C in the presence of 0.01% merthiolate. ⚠

5 For each ml of Sepharose suspension, add 5 ml of 1 M ethanolamine. Leave for 2 h at RT. ☐2

6 Wash the Sepharose on the scintered glass filter by the addition and removal of 40 ml of 0.1 M $NaHCO_3$ 0.5 M NaCl pH 8.3, followed by a wash in 40 ml 0.1 M acetate buffer 0.5 M NaCl pH 4.0. Repeat this alternate low/high pH wash twice.

7 Wash the Sepharose three more times with 40 ml of 0.1 M $NaHCO_3$ 0.5 M NaCl pH 8.3. ④

Pause points

☐1 Can also be left overnight at 4°C.

☐2 Can also be left overnight at 4°C.

Protocol 26. Ligand immobilization on Sepharose beads

Protocol 27. Immunoaffinity chromatography on columns

Reagents

Antibody or antigen solution to be purified
Elution buffer: 0.05 M diethylamine pH 11.5 ⚠
Ligand-coupled Sepharose (see *Protocol 26*)
1 M Phosphate buffer pH 6.8
Phosphate-buffered saline (PBS) pH 7.4

Equipment

Beakers (e.g. 100 ml and 1 liter)
Dialysis tubing, cellulose membrane
Empty PD-10 column (Pharmacia)
Fraction collector (optional)
Microcentrifuge
Microcentrifuge tubes
Peristaltic pump and tubing
Pipettes (e.g. 40–200 μl and 5 ml)
Pipette tips
UV monitor (spectrophotometer)

Technique

1 Cut the end off the tip of an empty PD-10 separation column. Ensure the sintered polyethylene frit is at the bottom of the column. Replace bottom cap. ①

2 Pour the ligand-coupled Sepharose into the column. ② 1

3 Remove the bottom cap and slowly add 5 ml of PBS to the top of the column, collecting the displaced fluid from the column into a waste beaker.

4 When all the PBS has entered the column by gravity, add 5 ml of elu-

Notes

① Alternatively construct a column from a 10 ml syringe barrel connected to a short length of rubber tubing (e.g. the syringe end from a butterfly needle), closed off by a clip. Pack the bottom of the column with glass wool.⚠ The top of the column will consist of the rubber stopper from the syringe plunger through which the butterfly needle has been inserted together with some of the attached tubing.

② These columns hold approximately 8.5 ml of Sepharose.

③ This procedure ensures that all material bound to the column is covalently linked and will not leach to any great extent

tion buffer to the top of the column, collecting the displaced fluid from the column into a waste beaker. ③

5 When all the elution buffer has entered the column by gravity, add 5 ml of PBS to the top of the column, collecting the displaced fluid from the column into a waste beaker.

6 Load 100 μl of antibody (or antigen) in PBS on to the column. ④

7 Pass PBS through the column using a peristaltic pump (1–2 ml/h) until all the unbound protein has been washed out. Collect the protein into microcentrifuge tubes. ⑤

8 Pass 0.05 M diethylamine pH 11.5 elution buffer through the column until the bound antibody (or antigen) has been removed. Collect the eluted protein in microcentrifuge tubes containing 1 M phosphate buffer pH 6.8. 1/20 the collection volume is normally sufficient for each tube. ⑥

9 Pass 20 column volumes of PBS through the column to re-equilibrate. [2]

10 Dialyze the eluted protein against several changes of PBS. [3]

11 Determine the protein concentration as described in *Protocol 1*.

from the column during the subsequent elution procedures.

④ The protein solution must be free of aggregated material or debris which can be removed by centrifugation at 10 000 *g* for 30 min. The binding capacity of the column, and hence the optimal concentration of antibody or antigen to be added, can be determined empirically.

⑤ The protein can be detected using a flow-through UV monitor or by collecting approximately 300-μl fractions and measuring the OD at 280 nm in a conventional spectrophotometer.

⑥ Elution can be monitored using a flow-through UV monitor or by collecting 300 μl fractions and measuring the OD at 280 nm in a conventional spectrophotometer. An alternative elution buffer is 0.1 M glycine-HCl pH 2.8 which may elute some proteins more efficiently than a high pH buffer. If eluting with the low pH buffer, collect into 1/20 the collection volume of 1 M phosphate buffer pH 8.0.

Pause points

[1] Store at 4°C with 0.01% merthiolate ⚠ in the buffer. Can be kept for many months.

[2] Columns can be stored for long periods of time (many months, often for years) at 4°C in buffer containing 0.01% merthiolate. They can be used many times without significant diminution of efficiency.

[3] Can leave dialyzing for 3–4 days in PBS containing 0.1% sodium azide. ⚠

Protocol 27. Immunoaffinity chromatography on columns

Protocol 28. **Batch immunoaffinity chromatography**

Reagents

Antibody
Diethylamine, 0.05 M pH 11.5 ⚠
Ligand-coupled Sepharose
1 M Phosphate buffer pH 6.8
Phosphate-buffered saline (PBS) pH 7.4

Equipment

Beaker (e.g. 1 liter)
Centrifuge (low speed benchtop)
Dialysis tubing, cellulose membrane
End-over-end rotary mixer (e.g. 10 r.p.m.)
Pipettes (e.g. 200–1000 μl)
Pipette tips
Test tubes (e.g. 55 × 11 mm)
UV spectrophotometer

Technique

1 Add 1 ml of antibody (or antigen) in PBS to 500 µl of ligand-coupled Sepharose gel.

2 Leave at RT for 2–4 h on an end-over-end mixer at slow speed. ①

3 Centrifuge the Sepharose at 300 g for 10 min.

4 Remove the supernatant and retain if required. ②

5 Resuspend the Sepharose in 1 ml of 0.05 M diethylamine pH 11.5 elution buffer. ③

6 Leave for 5 min at RT.

Notes

① Alternatively invert the tube by hand every 10–20 min during this period in order to mix the immunosorbent with the antibody solution.

② If purifying antibody from a polyclonal antiserum, once all antigen-specific reactivity has been removed the supernatant preparation can be used as an experimental control.

③ An alternative elution buffer is 0.1 M glycine-HCl pH 2.8 ⚠ which may elute some proteins more efficiently than a high pH buffer.

④ If eluting with 0.1 M glycine-HCl pH 2.8, neutralize with 1/20 the volume of 1 M phosphate buffer pH 8.0.

7 Centrifuge the Sepharose at 300 *g* for 10 min.

8 Aspirate the supernatant and immediately neutralize the eluted protein using 1/20 the volume of 1 M phosphate buffer pH 6.8. ④

9 Dialyze the protein against several changes of PBS. ☐1

10 Determine the protein concentration as described in *Protocol 1*.

Pause point

☐1 Can leave dialyzing for 3–4 days in PBS containing 0.1% sodium azide. ⚠

Protocol 28. Batch immunoaffinity chromatography

Immunoprecipitation (*Protocols 29 and 30*)

Immunoprecipitation followed by sodium dodecyl sulfate–polyacrylamide gel electrophoresis (SDS–PAGE) (*Protocol 31*) can be used to determine the presence, apparent molecular weight, and the approximate quantity of a specific protein present in a cell lysate or other complex mixture of antigens. A primary antibody provides the specificity whilst a secondary reagent mediates the precipitation step. Although anti-immunoglobulins can be extremely efficient precipitating agents, they are very sensitive to the ratio of anti-immunoglobulin to primary antibody in order that large enough complexes are formed for separation by centrifugation. Therefore, insoluble antibody-binding ligands such as *Staphylococcus aureus* Cowan 1 (SAC) or agarose beads coated with anti-immunoglobulin, protein A or protein G, are more commonly employed for the precipitation.

Protocol 29. Immunoprecipitation of liquid phase antigen

Reagents

Antibody specific for antigen of interest
Antigen solution
Protein A-coated agarose beads
50 mM Tris-HCl pH 6.8
62 mM Tris-HCl pH 6.8, 0.2% sodium dodecyl sulfate (SDS), ▽ 50 mM dithiothreitol ▲, 10% glycerol, 0.005% bromophenol blue
1% Triton X-100 ▲ in 0.1% bovine serum albumin (BSA) in 50 mM Tris-buffered saline (TBS) pH 7.5

Equipment

End-over-end rotary mixer
Microcentrifuge
Microcentrifuge tubes
Pipettes (e.g. 5–40 μl, 40–200 μl and 200–1000 μl)
Pipette tips
Water bath

Technique

1 Add 200 μl of antigen solution to 800 μl of TBS containing 1% Triton X-100 and 0.1% BSA. ①

Notes

① Antigen solution would be, for example, a complex mixture of antigens thought to contain the antigen of interest.

2 Add 5 μl of antigen-specific antibody. ②

3 Leave for 1 h at 4°C.

4 Add 50 μl of protein A-coated agarose beads. ③

5 Leave for 1 h at 4°C on an end-over-end mixer.

6 Centrifuge at 10 000 g for 15 sec.

7 Remove the supernatant and discard unless required for use as a control.

8 Resuspend the precipitated antigen in 1 ml of TBS containing 1% Triton X-100 and 0.1% BSA.

9 Centrifuge at 10 000 g for 15 sec.

10 Remove and discard the supernatant.

11 Repeat wash steps 8–10 three times but using 0.05 M Tris pH 6.8.

12 Remove and discard all the supernatant. For SDS–PAGE analysis resuspend in 20 μl of 62 mM Tris–HCl pH 6.8, 0.2% SDS, 50 mM dithiothreitol, 10% glycerol, 0.005% bromophenol blue.

13 Heat the sample in a boiling water bath for 3 min.

14 Centrifuge at 10 000 g for 15 sec.

15 Load the supernatant on to a reducing SDS–PAGE gel. ④

② A control tube should be set up in parallel using an irrelevant antibody (of the same class if monoclonal, same species if polyclonal). The optimal concentration of antibody may need to be determined empirically.

③ A less expensive alternative is to use fixed *Staphylococcus aureus* Cowan 1 (SAC). Although these often give good results they do sometimes give higher nonspecific binding compared with protein A-coated agarose beads.

④ See *Protocol 31*. Note that the heavy and light chains of the precipitating antibodies will be present (as bands of ~50 kDa and ~25 kDa) in addition to the precipitated antigen.

Protocol 29. Immunoprecipitation of liquid phase antigen

Reagents

Antibody specific for antigen of interest
Antibody that does not bind antigen of interest (control 'irrelevant' antibody)
Aprotinin ⚠
Cells containing antigen of interest
Phenylmethylsulfonyl fluoride (PMSF) ⚠ (100 mM stock in dried absolute ethanol)
Protein A-coated agarose beads
50 mM M Tris HCl pH 6.8
62 mM Tris–HCl pH 6.8, 0.2% sodium dodecyl sulfate (SDS) ⚠, 50 mM dithiothreitol ⚠, 10% glycerol 0.005% bromophenol blue ⚠
Triton X-100, 1% in 0.1% bovine serum albumin (BSA) in 50 mM Tris-buffered saline pH 7.5

Equipment

End-over-end rotary mixer
Microcentrifuge
Microcentrifuge tubes
Pipettes (e.g. 5–40 μl, 40–200 μl and 200–1000 μl)
Pipette tips
Ultracentrifuge
Vortex mixer
Water bath

Technique

1 Centrifuge 5×10^7 cells at 300 g for 7 min. ①

2 Remove and discard the supernatant.

3 Resuspend the cells in 1 ml 50 mM Tris-buffered saline pH 7.5 containing 1% Triton X-100, 0.1% BSA, 0.2 U/ml aprotinin and 1 mM PMSF (protease inhibitors).

Notes

① The procedure can be scaled up if using a larger number of cells.

② This preliminary centrifugation removes the cell nuclei.

③ Alternatively, but less ideally, microfuge at 10 000 g for 1 h.

④ This procedure pre-clears the lysate by removing proteins that bind nonspecifically to the anti-immunoglobulin or to

4 Leave for 1 h at 4°C.

5 Vortex the tube and then centrifuge at 300 g for 10 min. ②

6 Remove the supernatant and centrifuge this at 100 000 g for 30 min. ③

7 Remove the supernatant and add 5 μl of an irrelevant antibody to the supernatant. ④

8 Leave for 1 h at 4°C.

9 Add 50 μl of protein A-coated agarose beads. ⑤

10 Leave for 1 h at 4°C on an end-over-end mixer.

11 Centrifuge at 10 000 g for 15 sec.

12 Remove the supernatant and place in a clean microcentrifuge tube. Discard the tube containing the precipitate.

13 Add 5 μl of specific antibody to the supernatant.

14 Repeat steps 8–11.

15 Remove and discard the supernatant.

16 Resuspend the precipitated antigen in 1 ml 50 mM Tris-buffered saline pH 7.5 containing 1% Triton X-100 and 0.1% BSA.

17 Centrifuge at 10 000 g for 15 sec.

18 Remove and discard the supernatant.

Continued overleaf

protein A-coated agarose beads.

⑤ A less expensive alternative is fixed *Staphylococcus aureus* Cowan 1 (SAC). Although these often give good results they do sometimes give higher nonspecific binding compared with Protein A-coated beads.

⑥ See *Protocol 31*. Note that the heavy and light chains of the precipitating antibodies will be present (as bands of ~50 kDa and ~25 kDa) in addition to the precipitated antigen.

Protocol 30. Immunoprecipitation of cellular antigens

19 Repeat wash steps 16–18 three times but using 0.05 M Tris HCl pH 6.8.

20 Remove and discard all the supernatant. For SDS–PAGE analysis resuspend in 20 µl of 62 mM Tris–HCl pH 6.8, 0.2% SDS, 50 mM dithiothreitol 10% glycerol containing 0.005% of bromophenol blue.

21 Heat the sample in a boiling water bath for 3 min.

22 Centrifuge at 10 000 g for 15 sec.

23 Load the supernatant on to a reducing SDS–PAGE gel. ⑥

VI CHARACTERIZATION OF ANTIGEN OR ANTIBODY

There are a number of physical and biochemical features of an antigen that are relatively easy to characterize. An apparent molecular weight can be obtained using SDS–PAGE (*Protocol 31*) and the isoelectric point using isoelectric focusing (*Protocol 32*). Unless the antigen is pure, both of these techniques are likely to result in a large number of bands on the gel, only one (or a few) of which correspond to the antigen of interest. However, by transferring the separated proteins on to a solid support, such as a nitrocellulose membrane, the band(s) comprising the antigen of interest can be detected following the binding of a labeled antigen-specific antibody (*Protocol 34*).

Methods available

SDS–PAGE (see *Protocol 31*)

SDS covers proteins with a negative charge, the larger the protein the greater the charge. Thus, although the separation is due to charge, this will be related to the size of the protein. SDS–PAGE is often used to obtain an approximate molecular weight of a purified antigen. For impure antigens SDS–PAGE can be used in conjunction with immunoblotting [1–4].

Problems: Gives only an apparent molecular weight. The results are influenced by the ability of individual proteins to bind SDS and by post-translational modifications. Because the protein is denatured, discontinuous epitopes can usually no longer be detected by antibodies.

Isoelectric focusing (IEF; see *Protocol 32*)

This technique separates proteins on the basis of isoelectric point, thus pro-

References

1. Laemmli, U.K. (1970) *Nature* **227**, 680–685.
2. Hames, B.D. and Rickwood, D. (eds) (1990) *Gel Electrophoresis of Proteins: a Practical Approach*. 2nd edn. IRL Press, Oxford.
3. Weber, K. and Osborn, M. (1969) *J. Biol. Chem.* **244**, 4406–4412.
4. Patel, D. (1994) *Gel Electrophoresis: Essential Data*. John Wiley and Sons, Chichester.
5. Allen, R.C., Saravis, C.A. and Maurer, H.R. (1984) *Gel Electrophoresis and Isoelectric Focusing of Proteins*. Walter de Gruyter, New York.
6. Dunn, M.J. (1993) *Gel Electrophoresis: Proteins*. BIOS Scientific Publishers, Oxford.
7. Righetti, P.G. (1983) *Isoelectric Focusing: Theory, Methodology and Applications*. Elsevier, Amsterdam.

viding a pI value for the protein. Most commonly carried out in a polyacrylamide gel into which low molecular weight amphoteric compounds (carrier ampholytes) have been incorporated to produce a pH gradient. For impure antigens IEF can be used in conjunction with immunoblotting. IEF is also useful in the detection and characterization of different isoforms of an antigen. The technique can additionally be carried out as a preparative procedure in a liquid system [5–7].

Problems: The carrier ampholytes required to set up the pH gradient are fairly expensive. Post-translational modifications will influence the result

Immunoblotting (see *Protocols 34 and 35*)

The electrophoretic transfer of protein from a gel (SDS–PAGE, IEF, etc.) on to a solid support capable of binding protein, most frequently a nitrocellulose membrane. The membrane can then readily be probed with a labeled ligand to detect the transferred protein. Thus the technique can be used to ascertain the apparent molecular weight or the isoelectric point of a specific antigen amongst a mixture of proteins. A nonelectrophoretic version of the technique can be used to screen DNA expression libraries. Proteins are transferred to a nitrocellulose membrane directly from colonies of lyzed bacteria expressing the protein product of cloned DNA fragments [8–14].

Problems: Nitrocellulose membranes are fairly fragile and should be handled with care. High backgrounds can be a problem, but can often be reduced by using a different blocking agent and/or absorbing the antibodies used.

8. Burnette, W.N. (1981) *Anal. Biochem.* **112**, 95–203.
9. Gershoni, J.M. and Palade, G.E. (1983) *Anal. Biochem.* **131**, 1–15.
10. Towbin, H. and Gordon, J. (1984) *J. Immunol. Methods* **72**, 313–340.
11. Poxton, I.R. (1990) *Curr. Opin. Immunol.* **2**, 905–909.
12. Young, R.A. and Davis, R.W. (1983) *Proc. Natl Acad. Sci. USA* **80**, 1194–1198.
13. Bjerrum, O.J. and Heegaard, N.H. (eds) (1988) *Handbook of Immunoblotting of Proteins.* Vols. I and II. CRC Press, Boca Raton, FL.
14. Dunbar, B.S. (ed.) (1994) *Protein Blotting: a Practical Approach.* IRL Press, Oxford.
15. Geyson, H.M., Meloen, R.H. and Barteling, S.J. (1984) *Proc. Natl Acad. Sci. USA* **81**, 3998–4002.
16. Maeji, N.J., Bray, A.M. and Geyson, H.M. (1990) *J. Immunol. Methods* **134**, 23–33.
17. Rowlands, D.J. (1994) in *Synthetic Vaccines* (B.H. Nicholson, ed.), pp. 137–168. Blackwell Science Ltd, Oxford, UK.
18. Bodansky, M. and Trost, B. (eds) (1993) *Principles of Peptide Synthesis.* 2nd Edn. Springer-Verlag, New York.
19. Grant, G.A. (ed.) (1992) *Synthetic Peptides: a User's Guide.* W.H. Freeman & Co., New York.
20. Bidart, J.M., Troalen, F., Lazar, V., Berger, P., Marcillac, I., Lhomme, C., Droz, J.P. and Bellet, D. (1992) *Endocrinology* **131**, 1832–1840.
21. Becker, S., Armbruster, F.P., Muller, B., Echner, H., Kapurnotu, A., Livaniou, E., Mihelic, M., Stoeva, S. and Voelter, W. (1994) *J. Immunol. Methods.* **177**, 131–137.

Epitope mapping

To determine linear epitopes, overlapping peptides representative of the primary amino acid sequence of the protein of interest are synthesized on to polyethylene pins (PEPSCAN™, Cambridge Research Biochemicals) or cellulose membranes (SPOT™, Genosys) and then probed with antibodies [15–21].

Problems: Only continuous (linear) epitopes are detected using this technique. The majority of epitopes recognized by antibodies are discontinuous in nature, that is composed of amino acids that are not adjacent to each other in the primary sequence but which are brought together to form an epitope in the native protein, and thus are not fully detected by this technique. Note, however, that *part* of a discontinuous epitope may contain a linear stretch of amino acids which may bind the relevant antibody, albeit with weaker affinity than that seen with the full epitope. Once a representative peptide of a linear epitope has been identified, individual amino acids within the peptide can be substituted in order to define more accurately the critical residues. For approaches for mapping discontinuous epitopes see p. 8 (General Introduction: Characterization of antibodies).

Measurement of affinity

There are several methods available [22–27]. Among those commonly employed are:

1. Equilibrium dialysis. Only appropriate for small antigens (haptens) capable of diffusion out of a dialysis sac.

Protocols provided

31. *SDS-PAGE*
32. *Isoelectric focusing*
33. *Protein staining of SDS-PAGE and IEF gels*
34. *Immunoblotting*
35. *Antibody screening of DNA expression libraries*

22. Devey, M.E. and Steward, M.W. (1988) in *ELISA and Other Solid Phase Assays* (D.M. Kemeny and S.J. Challacombe, eds). John Wiley, Chichester.
23. Friguet, B., Chaffotte, A.F., Djavadi-Ohaniance, L. and Goldberg, M.E. (1985) *J. Immunol. Methods* **77**, 305–319.
24. Goldberg, M.E. and Djavadi-Ohaniance, L. (1993) *Curr. Opin. Immunol.* **5**, 278–281.
25. Stevens, F.J. (1987) *Mol. Immunol.* **24**, 1055–1060.
26. Seligman, S.J. (1994) *J. Immunol. Methods* **168**, 101–110.
27. Larsson, A. and Axelsson, B. (1991) *J. Immunol. Methods* **137**, 253–259.

2. Fluorescence quench. Measures the reduction in emitted fluorescence upon the binding of the antibody to the antigen.
3. Immunoprecipitation of bound labeled antigen over a range of antigen concentrations in antibody excess.
4. Competitive inhibition by fluid phase antigen of antibody binding to solid phase antigen.
5. Surface plasmon resonance (using the Pharmacia Biacore). Provides measurement of both on- and off-rates.

Problems: The figure obtained for the affinity of an antibody–antigen interaction varies depending upon the method used. However, most methods do provide a way of ranking antibodies in terms of their relative affinities. Surface plasmon resonance depends on the use of sophisticated and expensive equipment.

Choice of method

Depends on the information required. Immunoblotting can provide useful information with respect to multi-subunit antigens or antigenic fragments, for example following proteolytic cleavage. For the mapping of linear epitopes the PEPSCAN™ provides a good approach.

Separation and blotting of antigens (*Protocols 31–35*)

SDS–PAGE is usually carried out using a discontinuous system comprising a stacking gel into which the samples are initially electrophoresed, followed by a separation gel. Reference to the table below will indicate the percentage of acrylamide which is optimal for the resolution of various molecular size ranges.

Table 2. Composition of SDS–PAGE gels of different acrylamide percentages. The optimal separation range for each percentage is given in parenthesis

	6% (70–200 kDa)	8% (40–150 kDa)	10% (20–100 kDa)	12.% (10–70 kDa)	15% (8–50 kDa)
30% Acrylamide mix[a]	4.0 ml	5.3 ml	6.7 ml	8.0 ml	10.0 ml
10% Ammonium persulfate	200 μl	200 μl	200 μl	200 μl	200 μl
TEMED	16 μl	12 μl	8 μl	8 μl	8 μl
10% SDS	200 μl	200 μl	200 μl	200 μl	200 μl
1.5 M Tris pH 8.0	5.0 ml	5.0 ml	5.0 ml	5.0 ml	5.0 ml
Distilled water	10.6 ml	9.3 ml	7.9 ml	6.6 ml	4.6 ml

[a]30% acrylamide mix consists of 29.2% acrylamide and 0.8% N,N'-methylene-bis-acrylamide.

In the case of IEF gels, the carrier ampholyte mixture can be varied in order to obtain an optimal pI separation range for the proteins of interest. Once the proteins have been separated on either an SDS–PAGE or IEF gel, they can either be directly stained using Coomassie brilliant blue R, or be transferred on to nitrocellulose or nylon membranes for subsequent immunological detection. Even if the choice is immunoblotting, it is often desirable to stain the gel following transfer to confirm that all the proteins have been transferred. The trans-

Characterization of antigen or antibody

fer procedure is often referred to as Western blotting. Although nylon membranes are stronger and have a higher protein-binding capacity than nitrocellulose membranes, they generally give higher nonspecific binding of the detection antibodies. The electrophoretic transfer from gels to membranes can be carried out either as wet blotting in a tank full of buffer with vertically arranged wire or plate electrodes, or as a semi-dry transfer using a blotting cell with horizontal plate electrodes. The former is the more versatile approach, although semi-dry blotting provides rapid transfer with minimal buffer. It is also possible to immobilize proteins directly on to membranes without prior separation on gels. In this instance, whilst the protein can be simply spotted on to the membrane from a pipette, much more reproducible results are obtained if a microfiltration (dot-blot or slot-blot) unit is used. If necessary, the sensitivity of detection in immunoblots can be increased by using enhanced chemiluminescence in which the HRP-catalyzed oxidation of luminol is amplified and the emitted light detected using photographic film (e.g. using the ECL kit from Amersham).

Reagents

Acrylamide ⚠
10% Ammonium persulfate ⚠
Deionized distilled water
N,N'-methylene-*bis*-acrylamide ⚠
Molecular weight markers (Pharmacia)
Running buffer: 25 mM Tris, 190 mM glycine pH 8.3, 0.1% SDS
Sample in sample buffer: 62 mM Tris–HCl pH 6.8, 0.2% SDS ⚠, 50
  mM dithiothreitol ⚠, 10% glycerol, 0.005% bromophenol blue ⚠
Sodium dodecyl sulfate (SDS) ⚠
Stacking gel buffer: 0.5 M Tris–HCl pH 6.8, 0.4% SDS
N,N,N',N',-tetramethylethylenediamine (TEMED) ⚠
1.5 M Tris–HCl pH 8.0

Equipment

Beakers (10 ml and 50 ml)
Electrophoresis tank (e.g. Multiphor II, Pharmacia Biotech)
FlexiClamps (Pharmacia)
Glass gel plates
Gel comb
Microcentrifuge tubes
Pasteur pipettes
Pipettes (e.g. 5–40 μl, 40–200 μl, 200–1000 μl, 5 ml and 20 ml)
Pipette tips
Power pack
Spacers (0.5 mm)
Spatula
Staining dish
Stand and clamp
Water bath

Technique

1 Assemble two glass plates (e.g. 26 × 12.5 cm), separated from each
   other by a silicon rubber gasket (e.g. 0.5 mm thick). The gasket forms

Continued overleaf

Notes

① Minigel systems can also be employed.

② 30% acrylamide–*bis*-acrylamide mix can be purchased ready
   made. Wear disposable plastic surgical gloves when handling

a waterproof seal between the two plates which are held tightly together using FlexiClamps. Place the plates in a vertical position held securely using a stand and clamp. ①

2 Prepare 20 ml of the required percentage of separation gel (see *Table 2*, p. 103). After the acrylamide mix, SDS, Tris and distilled water have been mixed, add the ammonium persulfate followed immediately by TEMED. ②

3 Pour the acrylamide mixture between the two glass plates. Very carefully overlay the gel with 0.1% SDS, and leave at RT until polymerized. ③ ▢1

4 Following polymerization, remove the 0.1% SDS using a Pasteur pipette.

5 Prepare the stacking gel: 0.8 ml of 30% acrylamide mix in 2.95 ml of deionized distilled water and 1.25 ml of stacking gel buffer.

6 Add 15 µl of 10% ammonium persulfate followed immediately by 5 µl of TEMED. ②

7 Pour the stacking gel mixture on to the top of the polymerized separation gel.

8 Insert the comb and leave at RT until the stacking gel has polymerized after which the gel should be used as soon as possible. ④

9 Place the gel (still between the two glass plates) in the SDS–PAGE apparatus and add running buffer to the top and bottom reservoirs

acrylamide solutions. TEMED initiates polymerization and should, therefore, only be added immediately before pouring the gel.

③ Polymerization is complete after 0.5–2 h. Polymerization is indicated by the formation of a distinct interface between the overlay and the gel. It is often convenient to let the gel polymerize overnight.

④ Usually takes approximately 30 min.

⑤ Alternatively the gel can be stained directly as in *Protocol 33* to detect the protein bands.

10 In microfuge tubes, add 5 μl of 4 mg/ml sample to 20 μl of sample buffer.

11 Heat in a boiling water bath for 3 min.

12 Carefully remove the comb from the polymerized stacking gel, rinse the wells out with running buffer, and load the samples into the wells.

13 Run the gel at 75 V until the bromophenol blue enters the separation gel, then increase to 150 V. Run until the dye front approaches the bottom of the gel.

14 Dismantle the apparatus and very gently prise apart the glass plates using a spatula.

15 Transfer the protein from the gel on to a nitrocellulose membrane as described in *Protocol 34*. ⑤

Pause points

[1] The gel can be left at this stage at 4°C for up to a week.

Protocol 32. Isoelectric focusing (IEF)

Reagents

Acrylamide ⚠
5% Ammonium persulfate ⚠ in double-distilled water (freshly made each time)
bis-acrylamide ⚠
Carrier ampholytes (e.g. Ampholine, Pharmacia Biotech)
1 M Orthophosphoric acid ⚠
1 M NaOH ⚠
1 M Sucrose
Urea

Equipment

Beakers (100 ml)
3MM chromatography paper (Whatman)
Electrophoresis wicks
Flat bed isoelectric focusing apparatus
FlexiClamps
Glass plates
pH meter (with micro-electrode)
Pipettes (e.g. 0.5–10 μl, 200–1000 μl and 1–5 ml)
Pipette tips
Power pack
Side-arm flask and rubber stopper
Silicon rubber gasket
Spatula
Stand and clamp
Vacuum pump

Technique

1 Dissolve 3.75 g acrylamide, 0.112 g bis-acrylamide, 13.5 g urea and 9.0 g of sucrose in deionized double-distilled water to a final volume of 75 ml. ①

2 De-gas the acrylamide mixture using a vacuum pump and side-arm flask.

Notes

① Wear a protective mask and disposable plastic surgical gloves when weighing out acrylamide and bis-acrylamide.

② The glass plate is most easily removed from the gel by very gently prising apart with a large spatula.

3 Add 3.0 ml of carrier ampholytes covering the required pH range (e.g. pH 3.5–10).

4 Add 600 µl of 5% ammonium persulfate to 56.4 ml of the acrylamide mixture.

5 Pour the gel mixture between two 26 × 12.5 cm glass plates separated by a silicon rubber gasket and clamped vertically together with Flexiclamps. Leave at RT to polymerize. 1

6 Carefully remove the gasket and one of the glass plates. ②

7 Place the other glass plate with the gel uppermost on to a flat bed IEF apparatus following the manufacturer's instructions.

8 Soak the cathode wick in 1 M NaOH and place on one end of the gel so as to make contact with the cathode wire.

9 Soak the anode wick in 1 M orthophosphoric acid and place on the other end of the gel so as to make contact with the anode wire.

10 Pre-focus the gel at 15 W, 20 mA for 30 min.

11 Load the samples on to small squares (~0.5 × 0.5 cm) of 3MM paper placed in a row on the surface of the gel, parallel to the electrodes.

12 Focus the samples at 15 W constant power, 20 mA maximum, 1200 V. Run the gel for 1 h after the voltage reaches 1200 V.

Continued overleaf

③ Press the electrode gently against the gel and measure the pH at 0.5 cm intervals. Alternatively, standard marker proteins of known pI values are commercially available and can be focused on the gel at the same time as the samples.

④ Alternatively the gel can be directly stained as in *Protocol 33* to detect the protein bands.

Protocol 32. Isoelectric focusing (IEF)

13 Measure the pH gradient using a micro-electrode attached to a pH meter. ③

14 Transfer the protein from the gel on to a nitrocellulose membrane as described in *Protocol 34*. ④

Pause point

1. Following polymerization the gel can be kept at 4°C for several days.

Reagents

Acetic acid, glacial ⚠
Coomassie brilliant blue R
Distilled water
Methanol ⚠

Equipment

Orbital shaker
Staining dish

Technique

1 Submerge the electrophoresis gel in a tray containing 50% methanol 10% acetic acid in double-distilled water. Place on an orbital shaker and agitate gently for 2 h. ① 1

2 Pour off fixing solution and replace with 0.1% Coomassie brilliant blue R in 50% methanol 10% acetic acid, continue gentle shaking for 1 h.

3 Pour off the staining solution and rinse the gel with 50% methanol 10% acetic acid in double-distilled water.

4 Pour off the rinse solution and replace with 12% methanol 7% acetic acid (destain). Continue gentle agitation for 1 h.

5 Pour off the destain solution and replace with fresh destain solution. Continue gentle agitation until the gel becomes clear but the protein bands are still stained.

6 Examine the gel for stained protein bands. ②

Notes

① Be careful not to agitate too forcefully as this will cause the gel to break.

② IgG heavy chain has a molecular weight of ~50 kDa and Ig light chain ~25 kDa on SDS–PAGE gels. The gel may be placed on Whatman 3MM paper and dried using a vacuum gel drying apparatus if a permanent record is required. The wet gel can be stored in clingfilm at 4°C for 1–2 days and photographed.

Pause point

1 The gel can be fixed overnight if desired.

111

Protocol 34. **Immunoblotting**

Reagents

1% Bovine serum albumin (BSA), in TBS (blocking agent)
Diaminobenzidine (DAB) ⚠
Distilled water
Gel (SDS–PAGE or IEF) to be blotted
Horseradish peroxidase (HRP)-labeled anti-immunoglobulin
30% Hydrogen peroxide ⚠
Primary antibody to antigen of interest
Tris-buffered saline (TBS), 50 mM pH 7.5
TBS-T: 0.05% Tween 20 in TBS
Transfer buffer: 25 mM Tris, 192 mM glycine, 20% methanol ⚠ pH 8.3
  for SDS–PAGE gels and native gels containing acidic or neutral pro-
  teins. For IEF gels, native gels containing basic proteins, and acid urea
  gels the transfer buffer should be 0.7% glacial acetic acid ⚠

Equipment

Blotting tank and cassette
3MM chromatography paper (Whatman)
Nitrocellulose membrane, 0.45 μm
Orbital shaker
Plastic dishes
Power pack

Technique

1 Cut 0.45 μm nitrocellulose blotting membrane to the size of the gel. ①

2 Soak the membrane in the transfer buffer for 2–3 min. ②

3 Cut two pieces of 3MM paper to the same size as the gel.

4 Fill the blotting tank with transfer buffer.

5 Wet the 3MM paper, and the fiber pads from the blotting tank cassette,

Notes

① Handle carefully as nitrocellulose breaks easily.

② Carefully slide the membrane into the buffer at a 45° angle
to avoid trapping any air bubbles under the membrane. It is
essential that the entire membrane changes appearance
slightly when it becomes wet. If this should fail to happen
the membrane should be discarded and a fresh membrane
used. Handle with gloved hands to avoid the transfer of
grease or protein on to the membrane.

in transfer buffer.

6 Assemble the components into a sandwich using the tank cassette. ③

7 Place the sandwich cassette in the blotting tank, with the gel on the cathode side and the membrane on the anode side, or the other way round when using 0.7% glacial acetic acid transfer buffer.

8 Blot overnight at 30 V, 100 mA, or 30 V 200 mA when using 0.7% glacial acetic acid.

9 Remove the sandwich cassette from the tank and disassemble. Carefully peel the nitrocellulose membrane from the gel and place the membrane in TBS.

10 Wash the membrane in a dish of TBS at RT on an orbital shaker for 10 min. ④ 1

11 Transfer the membrane to 1% BSA in TBS at RT on an orbital shaker for 1 h. ⑤ 2

12 Wash the membrane twice in TBS-T for 5 min/wash.

13 Incubate the membrane with 10 mls of a predetermined optimal dilution of primary antibody in 1% BSA in TBS-T for 2 h at RT. ⑥

14 Wash the membrane three times in TBS-T for 5 min/wash.

Continued overleaf

③ The sandwich comprises: fiber pad, 3MM paper, gel, membrane, 3MM paper, fiber pad. It is essential that the gel and the membrane are in intimate contact throughout their entire surface area. This can be achieved by gently lowering the membrane on to the gel at an angle from one edge to the opposite edge and then rolling a glass rod over the membrane in order to squeeze out any residual air bubbles. Cut off one small corner from the gel and membrane to aid orientation.

④ All washes and incubation steps should be carried out on a gently rotating orbital shaker. NB The membrane will break up if the shaking is too vigorous.

⑤ This blocks unreacted sites on the membrane. Alternative blocking agents include 3% gelatin (heated to 50°C to dissolve), 3% hemoglobin, or 5% nonfat powdered milk (e.g. Marvel) in TBS.

⑥ The actual volume may vary depending on the size of the membrane but should be sufficient to cover the whole surface. This may be best achieved by sealing the membrane and the reagent in a plastic bag, but beware of air bubbles.

⑦ 5 mg DAB in 10 ml TBS with 10 μl of 30% H_2O_2 added immediately prior to use.

⑧ The color tends to fade upon drying and therefore the membrane is best photographed before it is dried.

Protocol 34. Immunoblotting

15 Incubate the membrane with 10 ml of a predetermined optimal dilution of HRP-conjugated anti-immunoglobulin in 1% BSA in TBS-T for 2 h at RT. ⑥

16 Wash the membrane twice in TBS-T, then twice in TBS for 5 min/wash.

17 Incubate the membrane in 10 ml of enzyme substrate in TBS at RT in the dark until color develops (usually within a few min). ⑦

18 Wash the membrane twice in distilled water for 5 min/wash.

19 Dry the membrane between two sheets of 3MM paper. ⑧

Pause points

1 The membrane can be kept at 4°C in TBS containing 0.1% sodium azide ⚠ for several days if necessary.

2 The membrane can be kept at 4°C in blocking agent containing 0.1% sodium azide for several days if necessary

Protocol 35. Antibody screening of DNA expression libraries

Reagents

LB-agar plates: 15 g Bacto-agar added to 1 liter LB medium and auto-claved, 50 μg/ml (final concentration) ampicillin added to the cooled agar immediately before pouring the plates

Bovine serum albumin (BSA), 1% in TBS

Diaminobenzidine tetrahydrochloride (DAB) ⚠

E. coli Y1090

Horseradish peroxidase (HRP)-labeled anti-immunoglobulin

30% Hydrogen peroxide (H_2O_2) ⚠

Indian Ink

Isopropyl β-D-thiogalactopyranoside (IPTG) ⚠ , 10 mM in distilled water

LB (Luria-Bertani) medium: 10 g Bacto-tryptone, 5 g Bacto-yeast extract, 5 g NaCl in 1 liter distilled water, autoclaved

10 mM $MgCl_2$, 10 mM Tris–HCl pH 7.5

Maltose

λgt 11 phage library

Primary antibody against antigen of interest

50 mM Tris-buffered saline (TBS) pH 7.5

TBS-T, 0.05% Tween 20 in TBS

Top agar: 0.8 g Bacto-agar in 100 ml LB medium, autoclaved, and then 1 ml sterile 1 M $MgSO_4$ added

Equipment

Dishes (e.g. 2 liter Pyrex)

Fluted flask (100 ml)

Incubator (37°C and 42°C)

Needles

Nitrocellulose membranes, 0.45 μm

Orbital shaker

Orbital shaking incubator (37°C)

Pasteur pipettes

Plates, 100 mm diameter (polystyrene)

Test tubes (e.g. 5 ml)

Tooth picks

Vortex mixer

Continued overleaf

Protocol 35. Antibody screening of DNA expression libraries

Technique

1. Streak out E. coli Y1090 *hsdR* on an LB agar plate and grow overnight at 37°C. ① ⬛1

2. Pick a single colony with a sterile tooth pick and grow in 10 ml LB medium, containing 50 μg/ml ampicillin and 0.2% maltose, to saturation (OD_{600} 2.0) at 37°C in a fluted flask with vigorous agitation.

3. For each 100 mm plate on to which the library is to be spread, add 200 μl of bacterial culture to 3×10^4 plaque-forming units of λgt11 phage library in 100 μl of 10 mM $MgCl_2$, 10 mM Tris–HCl pH 7.5 in a sterile test tube.

4. Incubate the test tube at RT for 20 min.

5. Add 2.5 ml of molten LB top agar at 45°C to 300 μl of phage-infected bacteria, swirl gently to mix, and pour on to a 100 mm LB agar plate.

6. Incubate the plates at 42°C for 4 h.

7. Carefully overlay the plates with dry IPTG-impregnated nitrocellulose membranes. ②

8. Incubate the membranes on the plates for 4 h at 37°C.

9. Stab a pattern through the nitrocellulose membranes and into the agar using a needle dipped in ink. ③

10. Carefully peel the membranes away from the agar. ④

11. Rinse the membranes in TBS-T for a few seconds. ⬛2

Notes

① All work involving recombinant DNA must be carried out in accordance with local and national guidelines governing the handling of such material.

② Soak the membranes in 10 mM IPTG for 10 min at RT and then allow to dry prior to use.

③ This is essential so that the location of the positive plaques on the agar plates can be determined later.

④ Duplicate membranes can be made by placing another membrane over the agar after the first membrane has been removed. Incubation can also be carried out overnight at 4°C.

⑤ This step blocks unreacted sites on the membrane. Alternative blocks include 3% gelatin (heated to 50°C to dissolve), 3% hemoglobin, or 5% nonfat powdered milk in TBS. Carry out all subsequent washes and incubations on a gently moving orbital shaker. Washes can be carried out in Pyrex dishes, incubations with smaller volumes in 100 mm polystyrene plates or sealed plastic bags.

⑥ In some instances primary and/or secondary antibodies can give high backgrounds due to binding to *E. coli* proteins. These reactivities can usually be removed by absorption of the antisera with *E. coli* cell lysates.

⑦ 6 mg of DAB in 10 ml of TBS with 10 μl of 30% H_2O_2 added immediately prior to use.

12 Incubate the membranes with gentle agitation in 1% BSA in TBS for 1 h at RT. ⑤ ③

13 Wash the membranes twice in TBS-T for 5 min/wash.

14 Incubate the membranes with 10 ml of an optimal dilution of primary antibody (against the antigen of interest) in 1% BSA in TBS-T for 2 h at RT. ⑥

15 Wash the membranes three times in TBS-T for 5 min/wash.

16 Incubate the membranes with 10 ml of an optimal dilution of HRP-conjugated anti-immunoglobulin in 1% BSA in TBS-T for 2 h at RT. ⑥

17 Wash the membranes twice in TBS-T, then twice in TBS for 5 min/wash.

18 Incubate the membranes in DAB in the dark until color develops. ⑦

19 Wash the membranes twice in distilled water for 5 min/wash. ④

20 Use the needle marks on the membranes to orientate them relative to the agar plates and, for putative positive plaques, remove a plug of agar using a Pasteur pipette.

21 Expel each agar plug from the Pasteur pipette into 1 ml of 10 mM MgCl₂, 10 mM Tris–HCl pH 7.5 and incubate for 1 h at RT with occasional vortexing.

22 Replate the phage-containing buffer and re-screen as above to identify individual clones. ⑧

⑧ This second round of screening is important in order to confirm individual positive clones.

Pause points

① The colony-containing plates can be stored at 4°C for 2–3 weeks if sealed with Nescofilm (Nippon Shoji Kaisha Ltd, Osaka, Japan).

② The membranes can be kept at 4°C for several days in TBS containing 0.1% sodium azide. ⚠

③ The filter can be kept for several days at 4°C in blocking agent containing 0.1% sodium azide.

④ The damp membranes can be wrapped in Clingfilm and kept for several days at 4°C.

Protocol 35. Antibody screening of DNA expression libraries

VII CELL DEPLETION AND ENRICHMENT

Although many methods for cell separation rely on the physical characteristics of the cells (for example, using density gradients, selective cell adherence, or phagocytosis of iron particles), antibodies provide cell-specific purification in a number of cell enrichment or depletion techniques.

Methods available

Density gradient centrifugation
A number of different types of gradients, both continuous and discontinuous, can be used for cell purification (e.g. Ficoll, Percoll, BSA, etc.) [1–4].
Problems: Straightforward but relies on buoyant density which may overlap between the cells of interest and other cell types. The cell yield from Percoll gradients may be quite low in some instances.

Adherence
Simple and cheap. Can give satisfactory results, especially for depletion of the adherent cells. In the presence of serum, monocytes/macrophages adhere to plastic or to Sephadex G-10, whilst monocytes/macrophages and B cells adhere to nylon wool columns [5–7].
Problems: By its nature rather nonspecific.

Fluorescence-activated cell sorter (FACS)
Single or multiparameter sorting is possible. Highly specific for the defined cell population [8–11].

References

1. Bøyum, A. (1968) *Scand. J. Clin. Lab. Invest.* **21**, Suppl. 97, 1–29.
2. Rickwood, D. (ed.) (1992) *Preparative Centrifugation*. IRL Press, Oxford.
3. Ford, T.C. and Graham, J.M. (1991) *An Introduction to Centrifugation*. BIOS Scientific Publishers, Oxford.
4. Gmelig-Meyling, F. and Waldmann, T.A. (1980) *J. Immunol. Methods* **33**, 1–9.
5. Hathcock, K.S. (1993) in *Current Protocols in Immunology* (J.E. Coligan, A.M. Kruisbeek, D.H. Margulies, E.M. Shevach and W. Strober, eds), pp. 3.2.1–3.2.4. Greene Publishing and Wiley-Interscience, New York.
6. Julius, M.H., Simpson, E. and Herzenberg, L.A. (1973) *Eur. J. Immunol.* **3**, 645–649.
7. Vujanovic, N.L., Rabinowich, H., Lee, Y.J., Jost, L., Herberman, R.B. and Whiteside, T.L. (1993) *Cell. Immunol.* **151**, 133–157.
8. Battye, F.L. and Shortman, K. (1991) *Curr. Opin. Immunol.* **3**, 238–241.

Problems: **Requires expensive and sophisticated apparatus.** Time consuming if large numbers of cells are required which constitute a minor proportion of the starting population.

Selection on antibody or antigen-coated plates (Panning) (see Protocol 36)

Simple and relatively quick technique in which antibody or antigen is coated on to a plastic surface in order to select the desired cell population [12–14].

Problems: Often much better for cell depletion (negative selection) rather than specific enrichment (positive selection).

Immunobeads (see Protocol 37)

Wide range of pre-coated beads available, including those with ligands for the capture of monoclonal antibodies, thereby permitting the generation of user-determined specificities [15–18].

Problems: Moderately expensive. For maximum efficiency it is important to optimize the bead:cell ratio which may be different for negative and positive selections.

Complement-mediated lysis (see Protocol 38)

Cells are incubated with complement-fixing specific antibody and then a source of complement is added to lyse the target cells [19–21].

Problems: Can only be used for cell depletion.

9. Omerod, M.G. (ed.) (1994) *Flow Cytometry: a Practical Approach*. 2nd Edn. IRL Press. Oxford.

10. Melamed, M.R. Lindmo, T. and Mendelsohn, M.L. (eds) (1990) *Flow Cytometry and Sorting*, 2nd Edn. Wiley-Liss Inc. New York.

11. Tanke, H.J. and van der Keur, M. (1993) *Trends Biotech.* **11**, 55–62.

12. Mage, M.G., McHugh, L.L. and Rothstein, T.L. (1977) *J. Immunol. Methods* **15**, 47–56.

13. Wysocki, L.J. and Sato, V.L. (1978) *Proc. Natl Acad. Sci. USA* **75**, 2844–2848.

14. Small, M. Majumdar, A.S., Liebermann, M. and Weissman, I. (1994) *J. Immunol. Methods* **167**, 103–107.

15. Pilling, D. Kitas, G.D. Salmon, M. and Bacon, P.A. (1989) *J. Immunol. Methods* **122**, 235–241.

16. Miltenyi, S. Muller, W. Weichel, A. and Radbruch, A. (1990) *Cytometry* **11**, 231–238.

17. Molday, R.S. and MacKenzie, D. (1982) *J. Immunol. Methods* **52**, 353–367.

18. Rasmussen, A.M. Smeland, E.B. Erikstein, B.K. Caignault, L. and Funderud, S. (1992) *J. Immunol. Methods* **146**, 195–202.

19 Hathcock, K.S. (1993) in *Current Protocols in Immunology* (J.E. Coligan, A.M. Kruisbeek, D.H. Margulies, E.M. Shevach and W. Strober, eds), pp. 3.4.1–3.4.3. Greene Publishing and Wiley-Interscience, New York.

20. Hunt, S.V. (1986) in *Handbook of Experimental Immunology* (D.M. Weir, L.A. Herzenberg, C. Blackwell

Choice of method

Immunobeads probably provide the best generally available method for both positive and negative selection of cell populations.

and L.A. Herzenberg, eds), Vol 2, Ch. 55. Blackwell Science, Oxford, UK.

21. Xia, M.Q., Hale, G. and Waldmann, H. (1993) *Mol. Immunol.* **30**, 1089–1096.

Protocols provided

36. *Cell selection on antibody or antigen-coated plates (Panning)*
37. *Cell purification using antibody-coated magnetic beads*
38. *Complement-mediated lysis of antibody-coated targets*

The following methods all rely on using the specificity of the antibody molecule to select a cell population on the basis of expression of a surface antigen, or to select B cells of a given antigen specificity. Not all cells of the desired population may express a given cell surface antigen at the same level and, therefore, there may be subpopulations that are not selected or cells may be contaminated with undesired cell types. For example, whilst CD5 is expressed on the majority of T cells, it is also found on a minor population of B cells. Likewise, CD4 is expressed not only on MHC class II-restricted T cells, but also on dendritic cells and on some human monocytes/macrophages. Cell populations should therefore always be defined by the marker used for selection, for example 'CD19+ B cells' rather than 'B cells'. If cells are subjected to positive selection, certain factors need to be considered. In particular, is it required that the selecting ligand be detached from the selected cells? Also, is it established beyond reasonable doubt that engaging the receptor recognized by the antibody does not lead to cell signaling, and if it does is this of relevance to the experiment?

Cell depletion and enrichment

Protocol 36. Cell selection on antibody or antigen-coated plates (Panning)

Reagents

Antibody or antigen
1% Bovine serum albumin (BSA), in PBS (blocking agent)
Cell suspension (⚠)
Medium (e.g. RPMI 1640 containing 2% heat-inactivated fetal calf serum (HIFCS) and antibiotics)
Phosphate-buffered saline (PBS) pH 7.4

Equipment

Centrifuge (low speed bench top)
Centrifuge tubes, 15 ml polypropylene
Hemocytometer
Ice bucket
Microscope
Petri dishes (60 mm diam., polystyrene)
Pipettes (e.g. 200–1000 μl and 1–5 ml)
Pipette tips

Technique

1 Place 2 ml of antibody or antigen at 10 µg/ml in PBS in to a Petri dish. Replace the lid and leave overnight at 4°C. ① ⓵

2 Wash the Petri dish three times with PBS.

3 Place 5 ml of 1% BSA in PBS in to the Petri dish. Replace the lid and leave for 1 h at RT.

4 Wash the Petri dish three times with PBS.

5 Add 5 ml of cells at 10^6/ml in medium containing 2% HIFCS and antibiotics. ②

6 Leave the cells in the Petri dish for 1 h at 4°C.

Notes

① Higher concentrations may give better results in some cases. All reagents and procedures in this protocol should be carried out under sterile tissue culture conditions.

② Cells may harbor human pathogens and should be handled accordingly in a class II microbiological safety cabinet. For cell samples from humans use only approved donors or persons previously screened for the absence of viral pathogens.

③ Alternatively the adherent cells can be removed by scraping with a rubber-coated rod.

④ The efficiency of the enrichment or depletion should be checked using immunofluorescence for relevant cell surface antigens.

7 Rinse the Petri dish very gently three times with cold medium (4°C) to remove nonbound cells. Keep the cells in a test tube on melting ice.

8 Vigorously wash the Petri dish by pipetting up and down with cold tissue culture medium (4°C) to remove the antigen-specific cells. ③

9 Centrifuge the antigen-specific and the nonantigen-specific cells at 300 g for 7 min.

10 Resuspend the cells in 500 µl tissue of culture medium and ascertain the cell concentration prior to further analysis. ④

Pause point

1 The Petri dishes can be left at 4°C for several days if the PBS contains 0.1% sodium azide ⚠ and the Petri dish is sealed with Nescofilm (Nippon Shoji Kaishi Ltd, Osaka, Japan).

Protocol 37. Cell purification using antibody-coated magnetic beads

Reagents

Buffer: 5% heat-inactivated fetal calf serum (HIFCS), 0.1% sodium azide ⚠ in PBS
Cell suspension (⚠)
Magnetic beads (e.g. Dynabeads) coated with anti-Ig (reactive with the primary antibody but not against the immunoglobulin of the species whose cells are being used)
Primary antibody to cell surface antigen of interest

Equipment

Centrifuge (low speed bench top)
Hemocytometer
Ice bucket
Magnetic separator
Microscope
Pipettes (e.g. 0.5–10 ul, 40–200 μl, 5 ml)
Pipette tips
Test tubes (e.g. 12 × 75 mm sterile polypropylene)
Vortex mixer

Technique

1 Centrifuge 10^7 cells at 300 g for 7 min at 4°C, aspirate the medium, and gently resuspend the cells in the residual medium using a vortex mixer.

2 Add 100 µl of a predetermined optimal concentration in buffer of the primary antibody against the cell surface antigen of interest.

3 Put the tube on melting ice for 30 min. [1]

4 Add 5 ml of cold buffer and centrifuge at 300 g for 7 min at 4°C.

5 Remove the buffer and resuspend the cells in residual buffer. Repeat

Notes

(1) For some purification procedures the magnetic beads can be used without prior incubation of the cells with primary antibody. For example, anti-mouse immunoglobulin-coated magnetic beads are suitable for direct isolation/depletion of murine B cells. Some magnetic beads (e.g. Dynabeads) are also available pre-coated with certain monoclonal antibodies, e.g. anti-CD19 for the purification of human B cells. Different bead:cell ratios may prove optimal in individual cases (e.g. 30:1).

(2) Although purpose-made apparatus may be purchased for this procedure, a powerful ordinary large magnet usually gives

the wash step twice by adding more cold buffer followed by centrifugation.

6 Resuspend the cells to give a final concentration of 5×10^6/ml.

7 Add anti-immunoglobulin-coated magnetic beads at a ratio of ~20:1
   beads:cells and keep at 4°C for 30 min. ①

8 Positively select cells by placing the tube against a magnet. ②

9 Remove the cells not retained by the magnet (negative population)
   whilst the tube is firmly attached to the magnet.

10 Remove the tube from the magnet to release the positively selected
   population. ③

11 Centrifuge negatively and/or positively selected cells at 300 g for 7 min
   at 4°C and resuspend at the desired concentration. ④

perfectly satisfactory results so long as the tube is securely
fastened to the magnet using Velcro or sticky tape.

③ If desired the beads can be removed by culturing the cells for
   10–20 h at 37°C in serum-containing medium. However, the
   efficiency of this procedure is very variable. Alternatively, in
   the case of some antibodies, a competing anti-Fab preparation can be used (DETACHaBEAD, Dynal) (see ref. 18,
   p. 119).

④ The efficiency of the enrichment or depletion should be
   checked using immunofluorescence for relevant cell surface
   antigens.

Pause point

1   Can be left overnight at 4°C.

Protocol 37. Cell purification using antibody-coated magnetic beads

Protocol 38. Complement-mediated lysis of antibody-coated targets

Reagents

Acridine orange ⚠ /ethidium bromide ⚠

Anti-immunoglobulin (reactive with primary antibody but not against immunoglobulin of the species whose cells are being used)

Buffer: 5% heat-inactivated fetal calf serum (HIFCS), 0.1% sodium azide ⚠ in phosphate-buffered saline (PBS)

Complement source (e.g. guinea pig serum, fresh or stored at –70°C)

Primary antibody against cell surface antigen expressed on the cells to be depleted

Equipment

Centrifuge

Hemocytometer

Pipettes (e.g. 0.5–10 μl, 200–1000 μl and 1–5 ml)

Pipette tips

12×15 mm round bottom test tubes

UV microscope

Vortex mixer

Technique

1 Centrifuge 10^6 cells at 300 g for 7 min at 4°C, remove the medium, and resuspend the cells in the residual medium using a vortex mixer.

2 Add 100 μl of a predetermined optimal concentration in buffer of the primary antibody against a cell surface antigen of the cells to be deleted.

3 Put the tube on melting ice for 30 min. [1]

4 Add 2 ml of cold buffer and centrifuge at 300 g for 7 min at 4°C.

5 Aspirate the buffer and resuspend the cells in the residual buffer. Repeat the wash step by adding more cold buffer followed by centrifugation.

Notes

(1) After this time take out 10 μl from the cell suspension, add this to 10 μl of acridine orange/ethidium bromide and determine the cell viability under a UV fluorescence microscope. Cells bearing the surface antigen for which the original monoclonal antibody was specific, should have been lyzed after this incubation period.

(2) Cell viability should be >95% because the complement-lyzed cells are removed by the wash steps. The efficiency of the depletion should be checked using immunofluorescence for relevant cell surface antigens.

6   Resuspend the cells in 100 µl of a predetermined optimal concentration in buffer of anti-immunoglobulin.

7   Put the tube on melting ice for 30 min.

8   Add 2 ml of cold buffer and centrifuge at 300 g for 7 min at 4°C.

9   Aspirate the buffer and resuspend the cells in the residual buffer. Repeat the wash step by adding more cold buffer followed by centrifugation.

10 Aspirate the buffer and add 1 ml of a predetermined optimal concentration of the complement source.

11 Incubate at 37°C for 30 min. ①

12 Add 2 ml of cold buffer to the cell suspension and centrifuge at 300 g for 7 min at 4°C.

13 Remove the buffer and resuspend the cells in residual buffer. Repeat the wash step twice more by adding more cold buffer followed by centrifugation.

14 Resuspend the cells in 500 µl of buffer and ascertain the cell concentration and viability prior to further analysis. ②

Pause point

1   Can be left overnight at 4°C.

Protocol 38. Complement-mediated lysis of antibody-coated targets

APPENDIX A: BUFFERS AND REAGENTS

0.1 M Acetate buffer, 0.5 M NaCl pH 4.0

1. Dissolve 8.2 g sodium acetate and 29.2 g NaCl in 900 ml double-distilled water.
2. Adjust pH to 4.0 with glacial acetic acid. △
3. Make volume up to 1 liter with double-distilled water.
4. Store at RT.

Acridine orange △/ethidium bromide △

1. Dissolve 1 mg acridine orange △ in 10 ml PBS (0.01% acridine orange stock solution).
2. Dissolve 2 mg ethidium bromide △ in 10 ml PBS (0.02% ethidium bromide stock solution).
3. Add 200 μl of each to 10 ml PBS.
4. Store wrapped in foil at 4°C.

Barbitone-buffered saline △, 0.15M pH 7.6 (5×)

1. Dissolve 5.75 g diethylbarbituric acid △ in 500 ml double-distilled water (heat to 95°C to dissolve).
2. Dissolve 85 g sodium chloride and 3.75 g sodium diethylbarbiturate △ in 1.4 liter double-distilled water and add to diethylbarbituric acid △ solution.
3. Dissolve 1.0 g $MgCl_2 \cdot 6H_2O$ and 220 mg $CaCl_2 \cdot 2H_2O$ △ in 5 ml double-distilled water, and add to above.
4. Make volume up to 2 liters with double-distilled water.
5. Store at 4°C.
6. Dilute 1 in 5 in double-distilled water for use.

Bicarbonate–saline buffer pH 7.4

1. Dissolve 8.4 g $NaHCO_3$ and 5.84 g NaCl in 900 ml double-distilled water.
2. Adjust pH to 7.4 with concentrated HCl.⚠
3. Make volume up to 1 liter with double-distilled water.
4. Store at RT.

0.025 M borate buffer pH 9.0

1. Dissolve 9.5 g sodium tetraborate decahydrate (borax) in 900 ml double-distilled water.
2. Adjust pH to 9.0 with 1 M HCl. ⚠
3. Make volume up to 1 liter with double-distilled water.
4. Store at 4°C.

Carbonate–bicarbonate buffer pH 9.5

1. Dissolve 8.6 g Na_2CO_3 and 17.2 g $NaHCO_3$ in 900 ml double-distilled water.
2. Make volume up to 1 liter with double-distilled water.

Buffer does not keep: make fresh buffer each time. (It is also possible to purchase carbonate–bicarbonate buffer capsules (for example from Sigma) which are simply dissolved in double-distilled water to produce the buffer.)

Coomassie brilliant blue R (0.05%)

1. Mix 40 ml double-distilled water, 50 ml methanol ⚠ and 10 ml glacial acetic acid. ⚠
2. Dissolve 50 mg Coomassie brilliant blue R in the above solution.
3. Store at RT.

0.05 M Diethylamine, pH 11.5 ⚠

1. Add 519 μl diethylamine ⚠ to 99.5 ml double-distilled water in a glass.
2. Adjust to pH 11.5 using concentrated HCl. ⚠
3. Prepare fresh each time.

Immunoblot transfer buffer

For SDS–PAGE gels and native gels containing acidic or neutral proteins: 25 mM Tris 192 mM glycine 20% methanol ⚠ pH 8.3 (3.0 g Trizma base, 14.4 g glycine in 1 liter of 20% methanol).

For IEF gels, native gels containing basic proteins, and acid urea gels: 0.7% glacial acetic acid ⚠ (7 ml in 993 ml double-distilled water).

LB medium

1. Dissolve 10 g Bacto-tryptone, 5 g Bacto-yeast extract and 5 g NaCl in 900 ml double-distilled water.
2. Make volume up to 1 liter with double-distilled water.
3. Autoclave.
4. Store at 4°C.

10 mM MgCl$_2$, 10 mM Tris–HCl pH 7.5

1. Dissolve 1.2 g Trizma base and 950 mg MgCl$_2$ in 900 ml double-distilled water.
2. Adjust to pH 7.5 with concentrated HCl. ⚠
3. Make volume up to 1 liter with double-distilled water.
4. Store at 4°C.

0.1 M NaHCO$_3$, 0.5 M NaCl pH 8.3

1. Dissolve 8.4 g Na$_2$CO$_3$ and 29.2 g NaCl in 900 ml double-distilled water.
2. Adjust to pH 8.3 with concentrated HCl. ⚠
3. Make volume up to 1 liter with double-distilled water.
4. Store at RT.

0.1 M NaHCO$_3$, 0.1 M NaCl pH 7.4
1. Dissolve 8.4 g NaHCO$_3$ and 5.8 g NaCl in 900 ml double-distilled water.
2. Adjust to pH 7.4 with concentrated HCl. ⚠
3. Make volume up to 1 liter with double-distilled water.
4. Store at RT.

1% Paraformaldehyde ⚠
1. Dissolve 10 mg paraformaldehyde ⚠/ml of warm (aids solubility) 0.15 M NaCl (8.7 g/l) pH 7.4.
2. Store at 4°C.

2% Paraformaldehyde, in 0.1 M phosphate buffer pH 7.4 ⚠
1. Dissolve 10 mg paraformaldehyde ⚠/ml of warm (aids solubility) 0.1 M phosphate buffer pH 7.4.
2. Store at 4°C.

1 M Phosphate buffer, pH 6.8
1. Dissolve 136 g KH$_2$PO$_4$ in 900 ml double-distilled water.
2. Adjust to pH 6.8 with 10 M NaOH. ⚠
3. Make volume up to 1 liter with double-distilled water.
4. Store at RT.

0.1 M Phosphate buffer, pH 7.4
1. Dissolve 13.6 g KH$_2$PO$_4$ in 900 ml double-distilled water.
2. Adjust to pH 7.4 with 10 M NaOH. ⚠
3. Make volume up to 1 liter with double-distilled water.
4. Store at RT.

Appendix A: Buffers and reagents

Phosphate-buffered saline (PBS) pH 7.4 (10×)

1. Dissolve 80 g NaCl, 2.0 g KCl, 11.5 g Na_2HPO_4 and 2.0 g KH_2PO_4 in 900 ml double-distilled water.
2. Check pH and adjust to 7.4 with 1 M NaOH ⚠ if necessary.
3. Make volume up to 1 liter with double-distilled water.
4. Store at RT.
5. Dilute 1 in 10 in double-distilled water for use.

(It is also possible to purchase PBS tablets or sachets of PBS powder (for example from Sigma) which are simply dissolved in double-distilled water to produce the correct buffer.)

SDS–PAGE running buffer (10×)

1. Dissolve 30 g Trizma base, 144 g glycine and 10 g sodium dodecyl sulfate ⚠ in 800 ml double-distilled water.
2. Make up volume to 1 liter with double-distilled water.
3. Store at 4°C.
4. Dilute 1 in 10 in double-distilled water for use.

SDS–PAGE sample buffer

1. Dissolve 3.8 g Trizma base and 1 g sodium dodecyl sulfate ⚠ in 400 ml double-distilled water.
2. Add 50 ml glycerol.
3. Titrate to pH 6.8 with concentrated HCl. ⚠
4. Add 3.9 g dithiothreitol ⚠ and dissolve.
5. Make up volume to 500 ml with double-distilled water.
6. Store at 4°C.

SDS–PAGE separation gel buffer
1. Dissolve 182 g Trizma base and 4.0 g sodium dodecyl sulfate ⚠ in 900 ml deionized double-distilled water.
2. Titrate to pH 8.8 with concentrated HCl.⚠
3. Make up volume to 1 liter with deionized double-distilled water.
4. Store at 4°C.

SDS–PAGE stacking gel buffer
1. Dissolve 30 g Trizma base and 2.0 g sodium dodecyl sulfate ⚠ in 400 ml deionized double-distilled water.
2. Titrate to pH 6.8 with concentrated HCl.⚠
3. Make up volume to 500 ml with deionized double-distilled water.
4. Store at 4°C.

0.1 M Sodium acetate, pH 6.0
1. Dissolve 13.6 g of sodium acetate (trihydrate) in 900 ml double-distilled water.
2. Adjust pH to 6.0 with glacial acetic acid.⚠
3. Make volume up to 1 liter with double-distilled water.
4. Store at 4°C.

1 mM Sodium acetate, pH 4.0
1. Dissolve 136 mg of sodium acetate (trihydrate) in 900 ml double-distilled water.
2. Adjust pH to 4.0 with glacial acetic acid.⚠
3. Make volume up to 1 liter with double-distilled water.
4. Store at 4°C.

10 mM Sodium phosphate saline, pH 7.0

1. Dissolve 1.64 g $Na_2HPO_4 \cdot 7H_2O$, 0.47 g $NaH_2PO_4 \cdot H_2O$, and 8.77 g NaCl in 900 ml double-distilled water.
2. Adjust to pH 7.0 with 1 M HCl ⚠.
3. Make volume up to 1 liter with double-distilled water.
4. Store at RT.

0.5 M Sodium phosphate buffer, pH 7.4

1. Dissolve 54.3 g $Na_2HPO_4 \cdot 7H_2O$ and 6.56 g $NaH_2PO_4 \cdot H_2O$ in 450 ml double-distilled water.
2. Make volume up to 500 ml with double-distilled water
3. Store at RT.

Top agar

1. Add 0.8 g Bacto-agar to 100 ml LB medium (see p. 130).
2. Autoclave to dissolve and sterilize.
3. Add 1 ml sterile 1 M $MgSO_4$.

50 mM Tris-HCL, pH 6.8

1. Dissolve 6 g Trizma base in 900 ml double-distilled water.
2. Adjust pH to 6.8 with 1 M HCl. ⚠
3. Make volume up to 1 liter with double-distilled water.
4. Autoclave and store at RT.

Tris-barbital buffer pH 8.6 (5×) ⚠

1. Dissolve 2.4 g barbital (5,5'-diethyl barbituric acid) ⚠ in 900 ml double-distilled water (heat to 95°C to dissolve).
2. Dissolve 44.3 g Trizma base in this solution.
3. Make volume up to 1 liter with double-distilled water.
4. Store at 4°C
5. Dilute 1 in 5 in double-distilled water for use.

50 mM Tris-buffered saline (TBS), pH 7.5

1. Dissolve 6.35 g Tris-HCl, 1.18 g Trizma base and 8.77 g NaCl in 800 ml double-distilled water.
2. Make volume up to 1 liter with double-distilled water.
3. Autoclave and store at RT.

APPENDIX B: SUPPLIERS

More complete listings of suppliers, together with the type of reagents or equipment available can be found in, for example, the Linscott's Directory of Immunological and Biological Reagents (8th edition 1994–1995, Santa Rosa, CA) or the Bio/Technology 1995 International Buyer's Guide (Bio/Technology Vol. 12, Special Issue). For example the Linscott's Directory lists 13 000 monoclonal and 14 000 polyclonal antibodies and their suppliers; whilst amongst the more than 1500 biotechnology companies listed in the Bio/Technology Buyer's Guide, there are over 200 suppliers of polyclonal and monoclonal antibodies. In the list below, country codes for phone and fax are omitted for North American (1) and UK (44) numbers, and are in parentheses for other countries. If phoning UK numbers from abroad the first 0 should be omitted. Where available, toll free (freephone) numbers have also been given (800 in North America, 0800 in UK).

Type of reagent or equipment	Suppliers include
General reagents, chemicals, etc.	Sigma-Aldrich-Fluka (SAF), Calbiochem, ICN
Antibodies	Aldrich, American Type Culture Collection, Amersham, Becton-Dickinson, Boehringer Mannheim, Calbiochem-Novabiochem, Cambridge Research Biochemicals, Chemicon, Coulter, DAKO, Dynatech, Harlan, Life Technologies (Gibco BRL), Organon, Peninsula, PharMingen, Serotec, Sigma, The Binding Site, Vector, Zymed
Electrophoresis equipment	Amersham, Applied Biosystems, Bio-Rad, E-C Apparatus, Heraeus, Hoefer Pharmacia Biotech, Jouan
Chromatography equipment	Amersham, Applied Biosystems, Bio-Rad, E-C Apparatus, Heraeus, Hoefer Pharmacia Biotech, Jouan
Nitrocellulose membranes, etc.	Amersham, Bio-Rad, Millipore, Schleicher & Schuell, Whatman

Centrifuges	Beckman, E-C Apparatus, Eppendorf, Heraeus, Hoefer Pharmacia Biotech, Jouan
Pipettes	Bibby Sterilin, Eppendorf, Gilson, Hamilton
Peptide synthesis	Chiron Mimotopes, Genosys
Glycobiology reagents	Oxford GlycoSystems, Dextra Laboratories
Tissue culture products	Corning Inc., Bibby Sterilin, Costar
Magnetic beads	Dynal, Calbiochem-Novabiochem

Accurate Chemical & Scientific Corp., 300 Shames Drive, Westbury, NY 11590, USA.
Tel 516 333 2221
Fax 516 997 4948

Aldrich Chemical Company, The Old Brickyard, New Road, Gillingham, Dorset SP8 4JL, UK.
Tel 0800 717181.
Fax 0800 378538.
1001 West St. Paul Avenue, Milwaukee, WI 53233, USA.
Tel 414 273 3830.
Fax 414 273 4979.

American Type Culture Collection, 12301 Parklawn Drive, Rockville, MD 20852-1776, USA.
Tel 301 881 2600/800 638 6597
Fax 301 816 4367

Amersham International Plc., Amersham Place, Little Chalfont, Bucks HP7 9NA, UK.
Tel 01494 544000.
Fax 01494 542266.

Amersham North America, 2636 South Clearbrook Drive, Arlington Heights, IL 60005, USA.
Tel 708 593 6300/800 323 9750.
Fax 800 228 8735.

Amicon GmbH, Neuer Weg 2, Witten D-58453, Germany.
Tel 2302 960600.
Fax 2302 800905.

Amicon Inc., 72 Cherry Hill Drive, Beverly, MA 21915, USA.
Tel 508 777 3622/800 343 1397.
Fax 508 777 6204.

Applied Biosystems GmbH, Brunnenweg 13, Weiterstadt D-64331, Germany.
Tel 6150 1010.
Fax 6150 101101.

Applied Biosystems, 850 Lincoln Center Drive, Foster City, CA 94404, USA.
Tel 415 570 6667.
Fax 415 572 2743.

Beckman Instruments (UK) Ltd, Oakley Court, Kingsmead Business Park, London Road, High Wycombe, Bucks HP11 1JU, UK.
Tel 01494 441181.
Fax 01494 447558.

Boehringer Mannheim Corporation, 9115 Hague Road, PO Box 50414, Indianapolis, IN 46250-0414, USA.
Tel 317 849 9350/800 428 5433.
Fax 317 576 2754.

Bibby Sterilin Ltd, Tilling Drive, Stone, Staffs ST15 0SA, UK.
Tel 01785 812121.
Fax 01785 813748.

Bio-Rad Laboratories Ltd, Bio-Rad House, Maylands Avenue, Hemel Hempstead, Herts HP2 7TD, UK.
Tel 0800 181134.
Fax 01442 259118.

Bio-Rad Laboratories Life Science Group, 2000 Alfred Nobel Drive, Hercules, CA 94547, USA.
Tel 800 4 BIORAD.
Fax 800 879 2289.

Calbiochem-Novabiochem (UK) Ltd, Boulevard Industrial Park, Page Road, Beeston, Nottingham NG9 2JR, UK.
Tel 01602 430840/0800 622935.
Fax 01602 430951.

Beckman Instruments Inc., 2500 Harbor Blvd, Fullerton, CA 92634, USA.
Tel 714 871 4848/800 742 2345.
Fax 800 643 4366.

Becton-Dickinson Europe, 5 Chemin des Sources, 38241 Meylan, France.
Tel 7641 6464.
Fax 7690 1965.

Becton-Dickinson, 2350 Qume Drive, San Jose, CA 95131, USA.
Tel 408 432 9475/800 223 8226.
Fax 408 954 2009.

Boehringer Mannheim UK Ltd, Bell Lane, Lewes, East Sussex BN7 1LG, UK.
Tel 01273 480444.
Fax 01273 480266.

Boehringer Mannheim GmbH, Sandhofer Str. 116, 68298 Mannheim, Germany.
Tel 6221 7591.
Fax 6221 7598509.

Calbiochem-Novabiochem Corporation, 10394 Pacific Center Court, San Diego, CA 92121, USA.
Tel 619 450 9600/800 854 3417.
Fax 619 453 3552/800 432 9622.

Cambridge BioScience, 25 Signet Court, Stourbridge Common Business Centre, Swann's Road, Cambridge CB5 8BR, UK.
Tel 01223 316855.
Fax 01223 60732.

Cambridge Research Biochemicals Ltd, Gadbrook Park, Northwich, Cheshire CW9 7RA, UK.
Tel 01606 41100.
Fax 01606 49366.

Cambridge Research Biochemicals Inc., Wilmington, DE 19897, USA.
Tel 302 886 5832/800 327 0125.
Fax 302 886 2370.

Chemicon International Ltd, 2, Bonnersfield Lane, Harrow HA1 2JR, UK.
Tel 0181 863 0415.
Fax 0181 863 0416.

Chemicon International Inc., 28835 Single Oak Drive, Temecula, CA 92590, USA.
Tel 909 676 8080/800 437 7500.
Fax 909 676 9209/800 437 7502.

Chiron Mimotopes Pty Ltd, 11 Duerdin Street, Clayton, VIC 3168, Australia.
Tel 3565 1111.
Fax 3565 1199.

Chiron Mimotopes, 4560 Horton Street, Emeryville, CA 94608-2916, USA.
Tel 510 601 3316/800 733 7025.
Fax 510 601 3300.

Corning Inc., PO Box 5000, Corning, NY 14831, USA.
Tel 607 974 0353/800 222 7740.
Fax 607 974 0292.

Costar UK Ltd, 10 The Valley Centre, Gordon Road, High Wycombe, Bucks HP13 6EQ, UK.
Tel 01494 471207.
Fax 01494 464891.

Dextra Laboratories Ltd, The Innovation Centre, The University, PO Box 68, Reading RG6 6BX, UK.
Tel 01734 861361.
Fax 01734 861894.

Dextra agent: V-labs, 423 North Theard Street, Covington, LA 70433, USA.
Tel 504 893 0533.
Fax 504 893 0517.

Difco Laboratories Ltd, PO Box 14B, Central Avenue, East Molesey, Surrey KT8 0SE, UK.
Tel 0181 979 9951.
Fax 0181 979 2506.

Difco Laboratories, PO Box 331058, Detroit, MI 48232-7058, USA.
Tel 313 462 8500/800 521 0851.
Fax 313 462 8517.

Dionex (UK) Ltd, 4 Albany Court, Camberley, Surrey GU15 2PL, UK.
Tel 01276 691722.
Fax 01276 691837.

Costar, 1 Alewife Center, Cambridge, MA 02140, USA.
Tel 617 868 6200/800 492 1110.
Fax 617 868 2076.

Coulter Ltd, Northwell Drive, Luton, Bedfordshire LU3 3BR, UK.
Tel 01582 567000.
Fax 01582 490390.

Coulter Corporation, PO Box 169015, Miami, FL 33116-9015, USA.
Tel 305 380 3800/800 526 7694.
Fax 305 883 6881.

DAKO Ltd, 16 Manor Courtyard, Hughenden Avenue, High Wycombe, Bucks HP13 5RE, UK.
Tel 01494 452016.
Fax 01494 441846.

DAKO Corporation, 6392 Via Real, Carpinteria, CA 93013, USA.
Tel 805 566 6655/800 235 5743.
Fax 805 566 6688.

Dionex Corporation, 1228 Titan Way, PO Box 3603, Sunnyvale, CA 94088-3603, USA.
Tel 408 737 0700.
Fax 408 739 4398.

Dynal (UK) Ltd, Groft Business Park, 10 Thursby Road, Bromborough, Wirral L62 3PW, UK.
Tel 0151 644 6555.
Fax 0151 645 2094.

Dynal International, PO Box 158, Skøyen, N-0212, Oslo 2, Norway.
Tel 2206 1000.
Fax 2250 7015.

Dynal Inc., 5 Delaware Drive, Lake Success, NY 11042, USA.
Tel 516 326 3270/800 638 9416.
Fax 516 326 3298.

Dynatech Laboratories Ltd, Daux Road, Billingshurst, West Sussex RH14 9SJ, UK.
Tel 01403 783381.
Fax 01403 784397.

Appendix B: Suppliers

Dynatech Laboratories Inc., 14340 Sullyfield Circle, Chantilly, VA 22021, USA.
Tel 703 631 7800/800 336 4543.
Fax 703 631 7816.

E-C Apparatus Corporation, 3831 Tyrone Boulevard North, St Petersburg, FL 33709-4198, USA.
Tel 813 344 1644/800 EC RANGE.
Fax 813 343 5730.

Eppendorf-Netheler-Hinz GmbH, Barkhausenweg 1, Hamburg, D-22339, Germany.
Tel 405 38010.
Fax 405 3801556.

Eppendorf North America Inc., 545 Science Drive, Madison, WI 53711, USA.
Tel 608 231 1188/800 421 9988.
Fax 608 231 1339.

Fluka Chemicals, The Old Brickyard, New Road, Gillingham, Dorset SP8 4JL, UK.
Tel 01747 823097/0800 262300.
Fax 01747 824596/0800 565750.

Gilson Medical Electronics (France) S.A., 72 Rue Gambetta, Villiers Le Bel, 95400, France.
Tel 3429 5000.
Fax 3429 5080.

Gilson Inc., 3000 West Beltline Highway, PO Box 62007, Middleton, WI 53562-0027, USA.
Tel 608 836 1551/800 445 7661.
Fax 608 831 4451.

Hamilton Bonaduz AG, PO Box 26, CH-7402 Bonaduz, Switzerland.
Tel 81 370101.
Fax 81 372563.

Hamilton Company, 4970 Energy Way, Reno, NV 89502-0012, USA.
Tel 702 858 3000/800 648 5950.
Fax 702 856 7259.

Harlan Bioproducts for Science Inc., PO Box 29176, Indianapolis, IN 46229, USA.
Tel 317 894 7536/800 9 SCIENCE.
Fax 317 894 1840.

Fluka Chemie AG, Industriestrasse 25, CH-9470 Buchs, Switzerland.
Tel 81 755 2511.
Fax 81 756 5449.

Fluka Chemical Corporation, 980 South Second Street, Ronkonkoma, NY 11779-7238, USA.
Tel 516 467 0980/800 FLUKA US.
Fax 516 467 0663.

Genosys Biotechnologies Inc., 162A Cambridge Science Park, Milton Road, Cambridge CB4 4GH, UK.
Tel 01223 425622.
Fax 01223 425966.

Genosys Biotechnologies Inc., 1442 Lake Front Circle, Suite 185, The Woodlands, TX 77380-3600, USA.
Tel 713 363 2212/800 234 5362.
Fax 713 363 2212.

Gilson Products, Anachem Ltd, 20 Charles Street, Luton, Beds LU2 0EB, UK.
Tel 01582 745000.
Fax 01582 483332.

Heraeus Equipment Ltd, Unit 9, Wates Way, Brentwood, Essex CM15 9TB, UK.
Tel 01277 231511.
Fax 01277 261856.

Heraeus Instruments GmbH, PO Box 1563, Hanau, D-63405, Germany.
Tel 6181 35413.
Fax 6181 35749.

Heraeus Instruments Inc., 111-A Corporate Boulevard, South Plainfield, NJ 07080, USA.
Tel 908 754 0100/800 441 2554.
Fax 908 754 9494.

Hoefer Pharmacia Biotech, Unit 12, Croft Road Workshops, Newcastle, Staffs ST5 0TT, UK.
Tel 01782 617317.
Fax 01782 617346.

Hoefer Pharmacia Biotech Inc., 654 Minnesota Street, PO Box 77387, San Francisco, CA 94107-0387, USA.
Tel 415 282 2307/800 227 4750.
Fax 415 821 1081.

ICN Biomedicals Ltd, Thame Business Park, Wenman Road, Thame, Oxfordshire OX9 3XA, UK.
Tel 01844 215522.
Fax 01844 213399.

ICN Biomedicals Inc., 3300 Hyland Avenue, Costa Mesa, CA 92626, USA.
Tel 714 545 0113/800 854 0530.
Fax 714 557 4872/800 334 6999.

Jouan Ltd, 130 Western Road, Tring, Herts HP23 4BU, UK.
Tel 01442 890202.
Fax 01442 891108.

Jouan S.A., Rue Bobby-Sands. C.P. 3203, 44805 Saint-Herblain Cedex, France.
Tel 40 949010.
Fax 40 947016.

Jouan Inc., 110-B Industrial Drive, Winchester, VA 22602, USA.
Tel 703 869 8623/800 662 7477.
Fax 703 869 8626.

Organon Teknika-Cappel, 100 Akzo Avenue, Durham, NC 27712, USA.
Tel 919 620 2000/800 523 7620.
Fax 800 432 9682.

Oxford GlycoSystems, Unit 4, Hitching Court, Blacklands Way, Abingdon, Oxon OX14 1RG, UK.
Tel 01235 553066/0800 212061.
Fax 01235 554701.

Oxford GlycoSystems Inc., Cross Island Plaza, 133-33 Brookville Boulevard, Rosedale, NY 11422, USA.
Tel 718 712 2693/800 722 2597.
Fax 718 712 3364.

Canberra Packard Ltd, 14, Station Road, Pangbourne, Berks RG8 7DT, UK.
Tel 01734 844981.
Fax 01734 844059.

Packard Instrument Company, 800 Research Parkway, Meriden, CT 06450, USA.
Tel 203 238 2351/800 323 1891.
Fax 203 639 2172.

Life Technologies Ltd (Gibco BRL), PO Box 35, 3 Fountain Drive, Inchinnan Business Park, Paisley PA4 9RF, UK.
Tel 0141 814 6100.
Fax 0141 887 1167.

Life Technologies Inc (Gibco BRL), 8717 Grovemont Circle, PO Box 6009, Gaithersburg, MD 20884-9980, USA.
Tel 301 840 8000/800 828 6686.
Fax 800 331 2286.

Millipore (UK) Ltd, The Boulevard, Blackmoor Lane, Watford, Herts WD1 2RA, UK.
Tel 01923 816375.
Fax 01923 818297.

Millipore Corporation, 80 Ashby Road, PO Box 9125, Bedford, MA 01730, USA.
Tel 617 275 9200/800 645 5476.
Fax 617 275 5550.

Organon Teknika Ltd, Cambridge Science Park, Milton Road, Cambridge CB4 4FL, UK.
Tel 01223 423650.
Fax 01223 420264.

Peninsula Laboratories Europe Ltd, Box 62, 17K Westside Industrial Estate, Jackson Street, St Helens, Merseyside WA9 3AJ, UK.
Tel 01744 612108.
Fax 01744 730064.

Peninsula Laboratories Inc., 611 Taylor Way, Belmont, CA 94002, USA.
Tel 415 592 5392/800 922 1516.
Fax 415 595 4071.

Pharmacia Biotech, 23 Grosvenor Road, St Albans, Herts AL1 3AW, UK.
Tel 01727 814000.
Fax 01727 814001.

Pharmacia Biotech AB, Björkgatan 30, S-751 82, Uppsala, Sweden.
Tel 18 165000.
Fax 18 143820.

Pharmacia Biotech Inc., 800, Centennial Avenue, Piscataway, NJ 08855-1327, USA.
Tel 908 457 8000/800 526 3593.
Fax 908 457 0557.

PharMingen, Cambridge BioScience, 25 Signet Court, Newmarket Road, Cambridge CB5 8LA, UK.
Tel 01223 316855.
Fax 01223 60732.

PharMingen, 10975 Torreyana Road, San Diego, CA 92121, USA.
Tel 619 792 5730/800 848 6227.
Fax 619 792 5238.

Schleicher & Schuell, Dassel, KR Northeim D-37582, Germany.
Tel 561 7910.
Fax 5561 791536.

Schleicher & Schuell Inc., 10 Optical Avenue, PO Box 2012, Keene, NH 03431, USA.
Tel 603 352 3810/800 245 4024.
Fax 603 357 3627.

Scotlab Ltd, Kirkshaws Road, Coatbridge, Strathclyde ML5 8AD, UK.
Tel 0236 449330
Fax 0236 449329

Sigma Chemical Company, 3050 Spruce Street, St Louis, MO 63103, USA.
Tel 314 771 5750/800 325 3010.
Fax 314 771 5757/800 325 5052.

The Binding Site Ltd, Birmingham Research Park, Vincent Drive, Birmingham B15 2SQ, UK.
Tel 0121 471 4197.
Fax 0121 472 6017.

The Binding Site Inc., 5889 Oberlin Drive, Suite 101, San Diego, CA 92121, USA.
Tel 800 633 4484.
Fax 619 453 9189.

Vector Laboratories Ltd, 16 Wulfric Square, Bretton, Peterborough, UK.
Tel 01733 265530.
Fax 01733 263048.

Vector Laboratories Inc., 30 Ingold Road, Burlingame, CA 94010, USA.
Tel 415 697 3600/800 227 6666.
Fax 415 697 0339.

Scotlab Inc., 30 Controls Drive, Shelton, CT 06484, USA.
Tel 800-SCOTLAB or 203 929-4038
Fax 203 929-7824

Serotec Ltd, 22 Bankside, Station Approach, Kidlington,
Oxford OX5 1JE, UK.
Tel 01865 379941.
Fax 01865 379941.

Serotec Ltd, Bioproducts for Science Inc., PO Box 29176,
Indianapolis, IN 46229, USA.
Tel 317 894 7536.
Fax 317 894 4473.

Sigma Chemical, Fancy Road, Poole, Dorset BH17 7NH, UK.
Tel 01202 733114/0800 373731.
Fax 01202 715460/0800 378785.

Whatman International Ltd, St Leonard's Road, 20/20
Maidstone, Kent ME16 0LS, UK.
Tel 01622 676670.
Fax 01622 677011.

Whatman Inc., 9 Bridwell Place, Clifton, NJ 07014, USA.
Tel 201 773 5800.
Fax 201 472 6949.

Zymed Laboratories Inc., 458 Carlton Court, South San
Francisco, CA 94080-9874, USA.
Tel 415 871 4494/800 874 4494.
Fax 415 871 4499.

INDEX

Nephelometry, 27
Nylon wool columns, 118

Ouchterlony, 26, 42

SDS-PAGE, 94, 99, 103–104, 105–107
   protein staining, 111
Selection
   negative, 119
   positive, 119

ESSENTIAL DATA SERIES

All researchers need rapid access to data on a daily basis. The *Essential Data Series* provides this core information in convenient pocket-sized books. For each title, the data have been carefully chosen, checked and organized by an expert in the subject area. *Essential Data* books therefore provide the information that researchers need in the form in which they need it.

Centrifugation
D. Rickwood, T.C. Ford & J. Steensgaard
0 471 94271 5   *March 1994   £12.95/$19.95*

Gel Electrophoresis
D. Patel
0 471 94306 1   *March 1994   £12.95/$19.95*

Light Microscopy
C. Rubbi
0 471 94270 7   *April 1994   £12.95/$19.95*

Vectors
P. Gacesa & D. Ramji
0 471 94841 1   *September 1994   £12.95/$19.95*

Human Cytogenetics
D. Rooney & B. Czepulkowski (Eds)
0 471 95076 9   *October 1994   £12.95/$19.95*

Animal Cells: Culture and media
D.C. Darling & S.J. Morgan
0 471 94300 2   *November 1994   £12.95/$19.95*

Cell and Molecular Biology
D. Rickwood & D. Patel
0 471 95568 X   *May 1995   £14.95/£23.95*

PCR
C.R. Newton (Ed.)
0 471 95222 2   *June 1995   £14.95/$23.95*

THE ESSENTIAL TECHNIQUES SERIES

The *Essential Techniques Series* provides accurate, up-to-date, quality information for the life scientist. These handy pocket-sized manuals are easy to carry, and conveniently spiral-bound making them ideal for lab bench work. *Essential Techniques* books provide value for money by giving all the information required in a single source.

Available in 1995 ...

Antibody Applications
P. Delves
0 471 95698 8   *September 1995*   *£14.95/$23.95*

Gel Electrophoresis of Nucleic Acids
P. Jones & D. Rickwood
0 471 96043 8   *October 1995*   *£14.95/£23.95*

PCR
J. Burke
0 471 95697 ·   *December 1995*   *£14.95/$23.95*

Forthcoming topics ...

Vectors: Cloning Applications
P. Gacesa & D. Ramjii

Vectors: Expression Systems
P. Gacesa & D. Ramjii

Gene Transcription
K. Docherty & J. Burke

Cell Culture
K. Brown

ORDER FORM

Please send me:

Qty   Title   Price/copy   Total

_____

_____

_____

_____

All prices are correct at time of going press but subject to change.

Your order will be processed without delay, please allow 21 days for delivery.

We will refund your payment without question if you return any unwanted book to us in a re-saleable condition within 30 days.

All books are available from your bookseller.

Method of payment

☐ Payment £/$ _____ enclosed (Payable to John Wiley & Sons Ltd).

Orders for one book only - please add £2.00/$5.00 to cover postage and handling. Two or more books postage FREE.

☐ Purchase order enclosed   ☐ Please send me an invoice
   (£2.00 will be added to cover postage and handling).

☐ Please charge my credit card account

☐ American Express   ☐ Diners Club   ☐ Visa   ☐ Mastercard

Card no: _____ Expiry date: _____

Signature: _____

Telephone our Customer Services Dept with your cash or credit card order on (01243) 829121 or dial FREE on 0800 243407 (UK only)

Send my order to:

Name (PLEASE PRINT) _____

Position: _____

Address: _____

_____

_____

_____

Telephone _____

Signature: _____ Date: _____

Return to:

Rebecca Harfield, John Wiley & Sons Ltd, Baffins Lane, Chichester, West Sussex, PO19 1UD, UK.

Fax: 01243 775878

or: Wiley Liss, 605 Third Avenue, New York, NY 10158-0012, USA

Fax: (212) 850 8888

☐ If you do not wish to receive mailings from other companies please tick
   this box or notify the Marketing Services Dept at John Wiley & Sons Ltd.

WILEY